INDIA BOOKVARSITY
LOTUS CHOICES
Editor: Mahendra Kulasrestha

Classics Revived
for an
Ultra-modern World

Learn RAJAYOGA from VIVEKANANDA

The first ever work in modern times
by a veteran

Yoga Explained
Patanjali's YOGA SUTRA
A Gallery of Asanas and
Selections on Yoga from
KURMA PURANA, SAMKHYA KARIKA,
SHVETASHWATARA UPANISHAD,
SHANKARA BHASHYA
and VYASA SUTRA

Published by

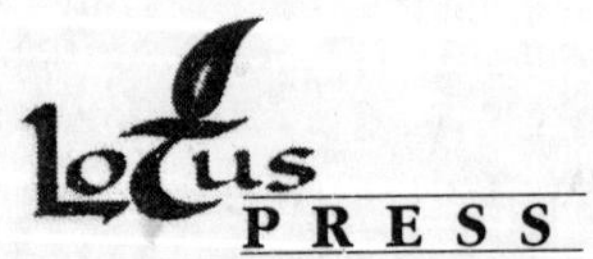

LEARN RAJA YOGA from Vivekananda

A grand exposition of India's unique philosophy and practice of Yoga, which Swami Vivekananda made for his American disciples

Lotus Press : Publishers & Distributors
Unit No. 220, 2nd Floor, 4735/22, Prakash Deep Building,
Ansari Road, Darya Ganj, New Delhi- 110002
Ph.: 23280047, 98118-38000
• E-mail : lotuspress1984@gmail.com
www.lotuspress.co.in

Source:
Swami Vivekananda's Writings
published by Advaita Asharam, etc.

Text out-of-copyright;
form, structure and notes; etc.
© Editor 2017

Learn Rajayoga from Vivekananda
© 2017, Lotus Press
ISBN: 81-8382-145-6

All rights reserved. No part of this publication may be reproduced, stored in a retrieval system, or transmitted, in any form or by any means, mechanical, photocopying, recording or otherwise, without prior written permission of the publisher.

Printed & Published by : **Lotus Press Publisher & Distributors,** New Delhi-02

Editorspeak

Pioneer in Modern Times

The credit of introducing as well as promoting the science and practice of Yoga—or Rajayoga to be more exact—to the West, America at the time, goes entirely to Swami Vivekananda. Along with the universalist Indian philosophy of Advaita or Vedanta, he presented to them Rajayoga as its second line management ideology, which helped in the actual attainment of the Brahman, or Godhead, however difficult it may be, was enthusiastically welcomed by his foreign disciples. The acquiring of good health was an added attraction. He therefore took regular classes, performed and lectured on the basic theories. He also translated the famous *Yoga Sutra* of Patanjali which propounded the complete eight-part practice in some detail. Needless to say, that all this was given to them in easy-to-understand English and in an idiom which suited them.

Vivekananda presented Rajayoga as a Science and not as a mish-mash of complicated philosophy. He compared its concepts with modern scientific theories, giving them an entirely different shape and look. This is one reason why Yoga spread in the West with such great speed. After him Swami Yogananda, Iyengar, and others took up the cause and gave it the shape of an all consuming tremendous movement—which it is today.

It is noteworthy—though sufficient attention has not been paid to it so far—that Vivekananda was working to give the whole philosophy and practice of Advaita and Yoga the organised shape and structure of a modern science. But he could not do so because of his very early demise—a most unfortunate event which enrages the present writer no end—it seems to him that gods do not support the really good and great people, why? Sister Nivedita in her writings, which are in no way inferior to her Master's, but have been ignored perhaps deliberately, throws definite and detailed light over this aspect of Swamiji's work.

Could all this work be taken up now?

It is therefore in the fitness of things that Vivekananda's work on this subject is being published in a properly organised form, with suitable emphases wherever required. It is easily the most authentic, complete and scientifically presented work on the subject in the plethora of books an Yoga coming out every day. Every Yoga enthusiast should give it a look in addition to whatever he takes recourse to in his practices.

Yoga is presently spreading like fire in America as well as Europe. Hundreds of centres are being run and gurus of all hues coming up. A few are trying to patent the ancient science and, no wonder, the acquisitive Western culture may grant such rights to some shameless grabbers.

But what is noteworthy and a matter of satisfaction is that some are involved in doing genuine research and expansion work in it to make it further useful to the modern man.

I would like to specially mention the work done by Debi Ross and Stuart Sovatsky in giving absolutely new dimensions to yogic practices. The former has succeeded in developing exercises connecting the physical with the mental, and the latter in making celibacy easier for the common man, youth in particular, who is uncontrollably driven to sex in modern times. His work, *Eros, Conciousness and Kundalini,* (published by Inner Traditions International, Rochester, Vermont 05176, U.S.A.) is a most revolutionary contribution to modern living worldwide, which, to my view, should be promoted in a suitable way. It is pleasant reading though the title sounds academic and does not express the real thrust of the book; it should be *Yoga for Celibacy in Modern Times.* Lovers will find it very useful and they will enjoy practising the new asanas. The price of the 212-page book is rather high.

There is further interesting news released by New York Times News Service, and published by the *Times of India* on 20 Oct. 05, that the Dalai Lama is for the past few years conducting research in meditation, on whether the intense meditation practised by monks can train to generate compassion and positive thoughts in them. Although some scientists are opposing such work, many neuro-scientists are actively supporting the new experiments. The Dalai Lama has been working with them to study how 'the practice of Buddhist contemplation affects moods and promotes a sense of peace and compassion.' In a study reported in 2003, Dr. Richard Davidson of the University of Wisconsin, led a team of 25 persons of a biotechnology firm, showed increased levels of mental activity in the left anterior temporal region of their brains after taking a course in meditation. This region is active during the sensations of happiness and positive emotion.

Dalai Lama has himself established an institute known as Mind and Life Institute for such research. In an investigation conducted with the help of Dr. Davidson, investigators tracked 'brain waves in eight Tibetan monks as they meditated in a state of "unconditional loving kindness and compassion". The researchers found that the monks were producing a very strong pattern of gama waves, a synchronised oscillation of brain cells that is associated with concentration and emotional control. A group of 10 college students who were learning to meditate produced a much weaker gama signal.'

With these and such other experimental efforts Yoga seems to have a still greater future. Let us use it 'Bahujana Sukhaya'—for the good of many.

Authorspeak

A Science like Physics

The old Sanskrit word Yoga is defined as '*chittavritti-nirodha*'. It means that yoga is the science that teaches us to bring the *chitta* under control from the state of change. The *chitta* is the stuff from which our minds are made and which is being constantly churned into waves by external and internal influences. Yoga teaches us how to control the mind so that it is not thrown out of balance into wave forms.

What does this mean? To the student of religion almost ninety-nine per cent of the books and thoughts of religion are mere speculations. One man thinks religion is this and another, that. If one man is more clever than the others, he overthrows their speculations and starts a new one. Men have been studying new religious systems for the last two thousand, four thousand, years—how long exactly nobody knows. When they could not reason them out, they said, "Believe!" If they were powerful, they forced their beliefs. This is going on even now.

But there are a set of people who are not entirely satisfied with this sort of thing. "Is there no way out?" they ask. You do not speculate that way in physics, chemistry, and mathematics. Why cannot the science of religion be like any other science? They proposed this way: If such a thing as the soul of man really exists, if it is immortal, if God really exists as the ruler of this universe—He must be known here; and all that must be realised in your own consciousness.

The mind cannot be analysed by any external machine. Supposing you could look into my brain while I am thinking, you would only see certain molecules interchanged. You could not see thought, consciousness, ideas, images. You would simply see the mass of vibrations—chemical and physical changes. From this example we see that this sort of analysis would not do.

Is there any other method by which the mind can be analysed as mind? If there is, then the real science of religion is possible. The science of Rajayoga claims there is such a possibility. We can all attempt it and succeed to a certain degree. There is this great difficulty: In external sciences the object is comparatively easy to observe. The instruments of analysis are rigid; and both are external. But in the analysis of the mind the object and the instruments of analysis are the same thing. The subject and the object become one.

External analysis will go to the brain and find physical and chemical changes. It would never succeed in answering the questions: What is this consciousness? What is your imagination? Where does this vast mass of ideas you have come from, and where do they go? We cannot deny them. They are facts. I never saw my own brain. I have to take for granted I have one. But man can never deny his own conscious imagination.

The great problem is ourselves. Am I the long chain I do not see—one piece following the other in rapid succession but quite unconnected? Am I such a state of consciousness for ever in a flux? Or am I something more than that—a substance, an entity, what we call the soul? In other words, has man a soul or not? Is he a bundle of states of consciousness without any connection, or is he a unified substance? That is the great controversy. If we are merely bundles of consciousness, such a question as immortality would be merely delusion.

On the other hand, if there is something in me which is a unit, a substance, then of course I am immortal. The unit cannot be destroyed or broken into pieces; only compounds can be broken up.

All religions except Buddhism believe and struggle in some way or other to reach such a substance. Buddhism denies the substance and is quite satisfied with that. It says, "This business about God, the soul, immortality, and all that—do not vex yourselves with such questions." But all the other religions of the world cling to this substance. They all believe that the soul is the substance in man in spite of all the changes, that God is the substance which is in the universe. They all believe in the immortality of the soul. These are speculations. Who is to decide the controversy between the Buddhists and the Christians? Christianity says there is a substance that will live for ever. A Christian says, "My Bible says so." A Buddhist says, "I do not believe in your book."

The question is: Are we the substance [the soul] or this subtle matter, the changing, billowing mind? Our minds are constantly changing. Where is the substance within? We do not find it. I am now this and now that. I will believe in the substance if for a moment you can stop these changes.

Of course all the beliefs in God and heaven are little beliefs of organised religions. Any scientific religion never proposes such things.

Yoga is the science that teaches us to stop the *chitta* [the mind-stuff] from getting into these changes. Suppose you succeed in leading the mind to a perfect state of yoga. That moment you have solved the problem. You have known what you are. You have mastered all the changes. After that you may let the mind run about, but it is not the same mind any more. It is perfectly under your control. No more like wild horses that dash you down. This is no longer a matter of speculation. There is no more Mr So-and-so, no more books or Vedas, or controversy of preachers, or anything. You have been yourself; I am the substance beyond all these changes. I am not the changes; if I were, I could not stop them. I can stop the changes, and therefore I can never be the changes. This is the proposition of the science of Yoga.

We do not like these changes. We do not like change at all. Every change is being forced upon us. In our country bullocks carry a yoke on there shoulders which is connected by a pole with an oil press. From the yoke projects a piece of wood to which is tied a bundle of grass just far enough to tempt the bullock, but he cannot reach it. He wants to eat the grass and goes a little farther, thereby turning the oil press. We are like these bullocks, always trying to eat the grass and stretching our necks to reach it. We go round and round this way. Nobody likes these changes. Certainly not! All these changes are forced upon us. We cannot help it. Once we have put ourselves in the machine, we must go on and on. The moment we stop, there is greater evil than if we continued forward.

Of course misery comes to us. It is all misery because it is all unwilling. It is all forced. Nature orders us and we obey, but there is not much love lost between us and nature. All our work is an attempt to escape nature. We say we are enjoying nature. If we analyse ourselves, we find that we are trying to escape everything and invent ways to enjoy this and that. Nature is like the Frenchman who had invited an English friend and told him of his old wines in the cellar. He called for a bottle of old wine. It was so beautiful, and the light sparkled inside like a piece of gold. His butler poured out a glass, and the Englishman quietly drank it. The butler had brought in a bottle of castor oil! We are drinking castor oil all the time; we cannot help it.

People in general are so reduced to machinery they do

not even think. Just like cats, dogs, and other animals, they are also driven with the whip by nature. They never disobey, never think of it. But even they have some experience of life.

Some, however, begin to question: What is this? What are all these experiences for? What is the Self? Is there any escape? Any meaning to life?

The good will die. The wicked will die. Kings will die, and beggars will die. The great misery is death. All the time we are trying to avoid it. And if we die in a comfortable religion, we think we will see Johns and Jacks afterwards and have a good time.

In the West they bring Johns and Jacks down to show you in seances. I saw such people a number of times and shook hands with them. They bang the piano and sing "Beulah Land": America is a vast land. My home is on the other side of the world. I do not know where Beulah Land is. You will not find it in any geography. See our good comfortable religion! The old, old moth-eaten belief!

These people cannot think. What can be done for them? They have been eaten up by the world. There is nothing in them to think. Their bones have become hollow, their brains are like cheese. I sympathise with them. Let them have their comfort! Some people are evidently very much comforted by seeing their ancestors from Beulah Land.

One of these mediums was offered to bring my ancestors down to me. I said, "Stop there. Do anything you like, but if you bring my ancestors, I don't know if I can restrain myself." The medium was very kind and stopped.

In our country, when we begin to get worried by things, we pay something to the priests and make a bargain with God. For the time being we feel comforted, otherwise we will not pay the priests. A little comfort comes, but it turns into reaction shortly. So again misery comes. The same misery is here all the time. Christian preachers in our country say, "If you believe in our doctrine you are safe." Our people among the lower classes believe in your doctrines. The only change is that they become beggars. But is that religion? It is politics— not religion. You may call it religion, dragging the word 'religion' down to that sense. But it is not spiritual.

Among thousands of men and women a few are inclined to something higher than this life. The others are like sheep. Some among thousands try to understand things, to find a way out. The question is: Is there a way out? If there is, it is in the soul and nowhere else. The ways out from other sources have been tried enough, and all have been found wanting. People do not find satisfaction. The very fact that those myriads of theories and sects exist show that people do not find satisfaction.

The science of yoga proposes this, that the one way out is through ourselves. We have to individualise ourselves. If there is any truth, we can realise it as our very essence. We will cease being driven about by nature from place to place.

The phenomenal world is always changing: to reach the changeless is our goal. We want to be that, to realise that Absolute, the changeless reality. What is preventing us from realising that reality? It is the fact of creation. The creative mind is creating all the time and gets mixed up with its own creation. But we must also remember that it is creation that discovered God. It is creation that discovered the Absolute in every individual soul.

Going back to our definition: yoga is stopping the *chitta*, the mind-stuff, from getting into these changes. When all this creation has been stopped—if it is possible to stop it—then we shall see for ourselves what we are in reality. The uncreated, the one that creates, manifests itself.

The methods of yoga are various. Some of them are very difficult; it takes long training to succeed. Some are easy.

Those who have the perseverance and strength to follow it through attain great results. Those who do not, may take a simpler method and get some benefit out of it.

As to the proper analysis of the mind, we see at once how difficult it is to grapple with the mind itself. We have become bodies. That we are souls we have forgotten entirely. When we think to ourselves, it is the body that comes into our imagination. We behave as bodies. We talk as bodies. We are all body. From this body we have to separate the soul. Therefore, the training begins with the body itself, until ultimately the spirit manifests itself. The central idea in all this training is to attain that power of concentration, the power of meditation.

The mind has a fine body and through this it works on the gross body. Vedanta says that behind the mind is the real self. It accepts the other two, but posits a third, the Eternal, the Ultimate, the last analysis, the unit, where there is no further compound. Birth is re-composition, death is decomposition, and the final analysis is where Atman is found; there being no further division possible, the durable is reached.

The whole ocean is present at the back of each wave, and all manifestations are waves, some very big, some small; yet all are the ocean in their essence, the whole ocean; but as waves each is a part. When the waves are stilled, then all is one; "a spectator without a spectacle", says Patanjali. When the mind is active, the Atman is mixed up with it. The repetition of old forms in quick succession is memory.

Be unattached. Knowledge is power, and by gaining one you get the other. By knowledge you can even banish the material world. When you can mentally get rid of one quality after another from any object until all are gone, you can at will make the object itself disappear from your consciousness.

Those who are ready, advance very quickly and can become yogis in six months. The less developed may take several years; and anyone by faithful work and by giving up everything else and devoting himself solely to practice can reach the goal in twelve years. Bhakti will bring you there without any of these mental gymnastics, but it is a slower way.

Ishwara is the Atman as seen or grasped by mind. His highest name is Om; so repeat it, meditate on it, and think of all its wonderful nature and attributes. Repeating the Om continually is the only true worship. It is not a word, it is God Himself.

Religion gives you nothing new; it only takes off obstacles and lets you see your self. Sickness is the first great obstacle; a healthy body is the best instrument. Melancholy is an almost insuperable barrier. If you have once known Brahman, never after can you be melancholy. Doubt, want of perseverance, mistaken ideas are other obstacles.

Pranas are subtle energies, sources of motion. There are ten in all, five inward and five outward. One great current flows upwards, and the other downwards. Pranayama is controlling the *pranas* through breathing. Breath is the fuel, *Prana* is the steam, and the body is the engine. Pranayama has three parts, Puraka (in-breathing), Kumbhaka (holding the breath), and Rechaka (out-breathing).

The Guru is the conveyance in which the spiritual influence is brought to you. Anyone can teach, but the spirit must be passed on by the Guru to the *shishya* (disciple), and that will fructify. The relation between *shishyas* is that of brotherhood, and this is actually accepted by law in India. The Guru passes the thought power, the Mantra, that he has received from those before him; and nothing can be done without a Guru. In fact, great danger ensues. Usually without a Guru, these yoga practices lead to lust; but with one, this seldom happens. Each Ishta has a mantra. The Ishta is the ideal peculiar to the particular worshipper; the mantra is the external word to express it. Constant repetition of the word helps to fix the ideal firmly in the mind. This method of worship prevails among religious devotees all over India.

The powers acquired by the practice of yoga are not obstacles for the yogi who is perfect, but are apt to be so for the beginner, through the wonder and pleasure excited by their exercise. *Siddhis* are the powers which mark success in the practice; and they may be produced by various means, such as the repetition of a mantra, by yoga practice, meditation, fasting, or even by the use of herbs and drugs. The yogi, who has conquered all interest in the powers acquired and who renounces all virtue arising from his actions, comes into the "cloud of virtue" (one of the states of Samadhi) and radiates holiness as a cloud rains water.

Meditation is on a series of objects, concentration is on one object. Complete continence gives great intellectual and spiritual power. The *Brahmacharin* must be sexually pure in thought, word, and deed. Lose regard for the body; get rid of the consciousness of it so far as possible.

Asana (posture) must be steady and pleasant; and constant practise, identifying the mind with the Infinite, will bring this about. Continual attention to one object is contemplation.

When a stone is thrown into still water, many circles are made, each distinct but all interacting; so is with our minds; only in us the action is unconscious, while with the yogi it is conscious. We are spiders in a web, and yoga practice will enable us like the spider to pass along any strand of the web we please. Non-yogis are bound to the particular spot where they are.

Contents

The Kingly Rajayoga

Patanjali's *Yoga Sutra*

Simple Lessons in Rajayoga

Rajayoga in Other Scriptures

I

The Kingly RAJAYOGA

Rajayoga in a Nutshell

A Summary from Kurma Purana

The fire of yoga burns the cage of sin that is around a man. Knowledge becomes purified and Nirvana is directly obtained. From yoga comes knowledge; knowledge again helps the yogi. He who combines in himself both yoga and knowledge, with him the Lord is pleased. Those that practise Mahayoga either once a day, or twice a day, or thrice, or always, know them to be gods.

Yoga is divided into two parts. One is called Abhava, and the other, Mahayoga. Where one's self is meditated upon as zero, and bereft of quality, that is called Abhava. That in which one sees the self as full of bliss and bereft of all impurities, and one with God, is called Mahayoga. The yogi, by each one, realises his Self. The other yogas that we read and hear of, do not deserve to be ranked with the excellent Mahayoga in which the yogi finds himself and the whole universe as God. This is the highest of all yogas.

Yama, Niyama, Asana, Pranayama, Pratyahara, Dharana, Dhyana, and Samadhi—are the steps in Rajayoga, of which non-injury, truthfulness, non-covetousness, chastity, not receiving anything from another, are called Yama. This purifies the mind, the chitta. Never producing pain by thought, word, and deed, in any living being, is what is called Ahimsa, non-injury. There is no virtue higher than non-injury. There is no happiness higher than what a man obtains by this attitude of non-offensiveness, to all creation. By truth we attain fruits of work. Through truth everything is attained.

In truth everything is established. Relating facts as they are—this is truth. Not taking others' goods by stealth or by force, is called Asteya, non-covetousness. Chastity in thought, word, and deed, always, and in all conditions, is what is called Brahmacharya. Not receiving any present from anybody, even when one is suffering terribly, is what is called Apartigraha. The idea is, when a man receives a gift from another, his heart becomes impure, he becomes low, he loses his independence, he becomes bound and attached.

The following are helps to success in yoga and are called Niyama or regular habits and observances: *Tapas*, austerity; *svadhyaya*, study; *santosha*, contentment; *shaucha*, purity; *Ishvara-pranidhana*, worshipping God. Fasting, or in other ways controlling the body, is called physical Tapas. Repeating the Vedas and other mantras, by which the Sattva material in the body is purified, is called study, Svadhyaya. There are three sorts of repetitions of these mantras. One is called the verbal, another semi-verbal, and the third mental. The verbal or audible is the lowest, and the inaudible is the highest of all. The repetition which is loud is the verbal; the next one is where only the lips move, but no sound is heard. The inaudible repetition of the mantra, accompanied with the thinking of its meaning, is called the "mental repetition", and is the highest.

The sages have said that there are two sorts of purification, external and internal. The purification of the body by water, earth, or other materials is the external purification, as bathing, etc. Purification of the mind by truth, and by all the other virtues, is what is called internal purification. Both are necessary. It is not sufficient that a man should be internally pure and externally dirty. When both are not attainable, the internal purity is the better, but no one will be a yogi until he has both. Worship of God is by praise, by thought, by devotion.

We have spoken about Yama and Niyama. The next is Asana (posture). The only thing to understand about it is leaving the body free, holding the chest, shoulders, and head straight. Then comes Pranayama. Praṇa means the vital force in one's own body, Ayama means controlling them. There are three sorts of Pranayama, the very simple, the middle, and the very high. Pranayama is divided into three parts: filling, restraining and emptying. When you begin with twelve seconds it is the lowest Pranayama; when you begin with twenty-four seconds it is the middle Pranayama; that Pranayama is the best which begins with thirty-six seconds.

In the lowest kind of Pranayama, there is perspiration, in the medium kind, quivering of the body, and in the highest Pranayama, levitaion of the body and influx of great bliss.

There is a Mantra called the Gãyatri. It is a very holy verse of the Vedas. "We meditate on the glory of that being who has produced this universe; may He enlighten our minds." Om is joined to it at the beginning and the end. In one Pranayama repeat three Gayatris. In all books they speak of Pranayama being divided into Rechaka (rejecting or exhaling), Puraka (inhaling), and Kumbhaka (restraining, stationary). The Indriyas, the organs of the senses, are acting outwards and coming in contact with external objects.

Bringing them under the control of the will is what is called Pratyahara or gathering towards oneself. Fixing the mind on the lotus of the heart, or on the centre of the head, is what is called Dharana. Limited to one spot, making the spot the base, a particular kind of mental waves rise; these are not swallowed up by other kinds of waves, but by degrees become prominent, while all the others recede and finally disappear.

Next, the multiplicity of these waves gives place to unity and one wave only is left in the mind. This is Dhyana, meditation. When no basis is necessary, when the whole of the mind has become one wave, one-formedness, it is called Samadhi.

Bereft of all help from places and centres, only the meaning of the thought is present. If the mind can be fixed on the centre for twelve seconds it will be a Dharana, twelve such Dharanas will be a Dhyana, and twelve such Dhyanas will be a Samadhi.

Where there is fire, or in water or on ground which is strewn with dry leaves, where there are many ant-hills, where there are wild animals, or danger, where four streets meet, where there is too much noise, where there are many wicked persons, yoga must not be practised. This applies more particularly to India. Do not practise when the body feels very lazy or ill, or when the mind is very miserable and sorrowful. Go to a place which is well hidden, and where people do not come to disturb you. Do not choose dirty places. Rather choose beautiful scenery, or a room in your own house which is beautiful. When you practise, first salute all the ancient yogis, and your own Guru, and God, and then begin.

Dhyana is spoken of and examples are now given of what to meditate upon. Sit straight, and look at the tip of your nose. This concentrates the mind, and by controlling the two optic nerves one advances a long way towards the control of the arc of reaction, and so to the control of the will. Here are a few specimens of meditation. Imagine a lotus upon the top of the head several inches up, with virtue as its centre, and knowledge as its stalk.

The eight petals of the lotus are the eight powers of the yogi. Inside, the stamens and pistils are renunciation. If the yogi refuses the external powers he will come to salvation. So the eight petals of the lotus are the eight powers, but the internal stamens and pistils are extreme renunciation, the renunciation of all these powers. Inside of that lotus think of the Golden One, the Almighty, the Intangible, He whose name is Om, the Inexpressible, surrounded with effulgent light. Meditate on that.

Another meditation is given. Think of a space in your heart, and in the midst of that space think that a flame is burning. Think of that flame as your own soul and inside the flame is another effulgent light, and that is the Soul of your soul, God. Meditate upon that in the heart.

Chastity, non-injury, forgiving even the greatest enemy, truth, faith in the Lord, these are all different *vrittis*. Be not afraid if you are not perfect in all of these; work, they will come. He who has given up all attachment, all fear, and all anger, he whose whole soul has gone unto the Lord, he who has taken refuge in the Lord, whose heart has become purified, with whatsoever desire he comes to the Lord, He will grant that to him. Therefore, worship Him through knowledge, love, or renunciation.

The Gita says of the yogi: "He who hates none, who is the friend of all, who is merciful to all, who has nothing of his own, who is free from egoism, who is even-minded in pain and pleasure, who is forbearing, who is always satisfied, who works always in yoga, whose self has become controlled, whose will is firm, whose mind and intellect are given up unto Me, such a one is My beloved *bhakta*. From whom comes no disturbance, who cannot be disturbed by others, who is free from joy, anger, fear, and anxiety, such a one is My beloved. He who does not depend on anything, who is pure and active, who does not care whether good comes or evil, and never becomes miserable, who has given up all efforts for himself; who is the same in praise or in blame, with a silent, thoughtful mind, blessed with what little comes in his way, homeless, for the whole world in his home, ane who is steady in his ideas, such a one is My beloved *bhakta*."

There was a great god-sage called Narada. Just as there are sages among mankind, great yogis, so there are great yogis among the gods. Narada was a good yogi, and very great. He travelled everywhere. One day he was passing through a forest, and saw a man who had been meditating until the white ants had built a huge mound round his body—so long had he been sitting in that position. He said to Narada, "Where are you going?" His mind and gestures were wild. Narada said, "I am going to heaven." "Then ask God when He will be merciful to me, when I shall attain freedom."

Further on, Narada saw another man. He was jumping about, singing, dancing, and said, "O Narada, where are you going?" His voice and gestures were wild. Narada said, "I am going to heaven." "Then, ask when I shall be free." Narada went on.

In course of time he came again by the same road, and there was the man who had been meditating with the ant-hill round him. He said, "O Narada, did you ask the Lord about me?" "O yes." "What did He say?" "The Lord told me that you would attain freedom in four more births." Then the man began to weep and wail, and said, "I have meditated until an ant-hill has grown around me, and I have four more births yet!"

Narada went to the other man. "Did you ask my question?" "O yes. Do you see this tamarind tree? I have to tell you that as many leaves as there are on that tree, so many times you shall be born, and then you shall attain freedom." The man began to dance for joy, and said, "I shall have freedom after such a short time!" A voice came, "My child, you will have freedom this minute."

That was the reward for his perseverance. He was ready to work through all those births; nothing discouraged him.

But the first man felt that even four more births were too long. Only perseverance like that of the man who was willing to wait aeons brings about the highest result.

1

A Systematic Method

All our knowledge is based upon experience. What we call inferential knowlege, in which we go from the less to the more general, or from the general to the particular, has experience as its basis. In what are called the exact sciences, people easily find the truth, because it appeals to the particular experiences of every human being. The scientist does not tell you to believe in anything, but he has certain results which come from his own experiences, and reasoning on them when he asks us to believe in his conclusions, he appeals to some universal experience of humanity. In every exact science there is a basis which is common to all humanity, so that we can at once see the truth or the fallacy of the conclusions drawn therefrom. Now, the question is: Has religion any such basis or not? I shall have to answer the question both in the affirmative and in the negative.

Religion, as it is generally taught all over the world, is said to be based upon faith and belief, and, in most cases, consists only of different sets of theories, and that is the reason why we find all religions quarrelling with one another. These theories, again, are based upon belief. One man says there is a great Being sitting above the clouds and governing the whole universe, and he asks me to believe that solely on the authority of his assertion. In the same way, I may have my own ideas, which I am asking others to believe, and if they ask for a reason, I cannot give them any. This is why religion and meta-physical philosophy have a bad name nowadays.

Every educated man seems to say, "Oh, these religions are only bundles of theories without any standard to judge them by, each man preaching his own pet ideas." Nevertheless, there is a basis of universal belief in religion, governing all the different theories, and all the varying ideas of different sects in different countries. Going to their basis we find that they also are based upon universal experiences.

In the first place, if you analyse all the various religions of the world, you will find that these are divided into two classes, those with a book, and those without a book. Those with a book are the strongest, and have the largest number of followers. Those without books have mostly died out, and the few new ones have very small followings. Yet, in all of them what they teach are the results of the experiences of particular persons.

The Christian asks you to believe in his religion, to believe in Christ and to believe in him as the incarnation of God, to believe in God, in a soul, and in a better state of that soul. If I ask him for reason, he says he believes in them. But if you go to the fountainhead of Christianity, you will find that it is based upon experience. Christ said he saw God; the disciples said they felt God; and so forth.

Similarly, in Buddhism, it is Buddha's experience. He experienced certain truths, saw them, came in contact with them, and preached them to the world. So is with the Hindus. In their books, the writers who are called Rishis, or sages, declare they experienced certain truths, saw them, came in contact with them, and preached them to the world. Thus, it is clear that all the religions of the world have been built upon that one universal and adamantine foundation of all our knowledge—direct experience.

The teachers all saw God; they all saw their own souls, they saw their future, they saw their eternity, and what they saw they preached. Only there is this difference, that by most of these religions, especially in modern times, a peculiar claim is made, namely, that these experiences are impossible at the present day; they were only possible with a few men, who were the first founders of the religions that subsequently bore their names. At the present time these experiences have become obsolete, and, therefore, we have now to take religion on belief.

This I entirely deny. If there has been one experience in this world in any particular branch of knowledge, it absolutely follows that the experience has been possible millions of times before, and will be repeated eternally. Uniformity is the rigorous law of nature, what once happened can happen always.

The teachers of the science of yoga, therefore, declare that religion is not only based upon the experience of ancient times, but that no man can be religious until he has the same perceptions himself. Yoga is the science which teaches us how to get these perceptions. It is not much use to talk about religion until one has felt it.

Why is there so much disturbance, so much fighting and quarrelling in the name of God? There has been more bloodshed in the name of God than for any other cause, because people never went to the fountainhead; they were content only to give a mental assent to the customs of their forefathers, and wanted others to do the same. What right has a man to say he has a soul if he does not feel it, or that there is a God if he does not see Him? If there is a God, we must see Him, if there is a soul, we must perceive it; otherwise it is better not to believe. It is better to be an outspoken atheist than a hypocrite.

The modern idea, on the one hand, with the "learned", is that religion and metaphysics and all search after a Supreme Being are futile; on the other hand, with the semi-educated, the idea seems to be that these things really have no basis; their only value consists in the fact that they furnish strong motive powers for doing good to the world. If men believe in God, they may become good, and moral, and so make good citizens.

We cannot blame them for holding such ideas, seeing that all the teaching these men get is simply to believe in an eternal rigmarole of words, without any substance behind them. They are asked to live upon words; can they do it? If they could, I should not have the least regard for human nature.

Man wants truth, wants to experience truth for himself; when he has grasped it, realised it, felt it within his heart of hearts, then alone, declare the Vedas, would all doubts vanish, all darkness be scattered, and all crookedness be made straight. "Ye children of immortality, even those who live in the highest sphere, the way is found; there is a way out of all this darkness, and that is by perceiving Him who is beyond all darkness; there is no other way."

The science of Rajayoga proposes to put before humanity a practical and scientifically worked out method of reaching this truth. In the first place, every science must have its own method of investigation. If you want to become an astronomer and sit down and cry "Astronomy! Astronomy!"—it will never is come to you. The same is with chemistry. A certain method must be followed. You must go to a laboratory, take different substances, mix them up, compound them, experiment with them, and out of that will come a knowledge of chemistry. If you want to be an astronomer you must go to an observatory, take a telescope, study the stars and planets, and then you will become an astronomer.

Each science must have its own methods. I could preach you thousands of sermons, but they would not make you religious, until you practised the method. These are the truths of the sages of all countries, of all ages, of men pure and unselfish, who had no motive but to do good to the world. They all declare that they have found some truth higher than what the senses can bring to us, and they invite verification. They ask us to take up the method and practise honestly, and then, if we do not find this higher truth, we will have the right to say there is no truth in the claim, but before we have done that, we are not rational in denying the truth of their assertions. So we must work faithfully, using the prescribed methods, and light will come.

In acquiring knowledge we make use of generalisation, and generalisation is based upon observation. We first observe facts, then generalise, and then draw conclusions or principles. The knowledge of the mind, of the internal nature of man, of thought, can never be had until we have first the power of observing the facts that are going on within.

It is comparatively easy to observe facts in the external world, for many instruments have been invented for the purpose, but in the internal world we have no instrument to help us. Yet we know we must observe in order to have a real science. Without a proper analysis, any science will be hopeless—mere theorising. And that is why all the psychologists have been quarrelling among themselves since the beginning of time, except those few who found out the means of observation.

The science of Rajayoga, in the first place, proposes to give us such a means of observing the internal states. The instrument is the mind itself. The power of attention, when properly guided, and directed towards the internal world, will analyse the mind, and illumine facts for us.

The powers of the mind are like rays of light dissipated; when they are concentrated, they illumine. This is our only means of knowledge. Everyone is using it, both in the external and the internal world; but, for the psychologist, the same minute observation has to be directed to the internal world, which the scientific man directs to the external; and this requires a great deal of practice.

From our childhood upwards we have been taught only to pay attention to external things, but never to internal things, hence most of us have nearly lost the faculty of observing the internal mechanism. To turn the mind, as it were, inside, stop it from going outside, and then to concentrate all its powers, and throw them upon the mind itself, in order that it may know its own nature, analyse itself, is very hard work. Yet that is the only way to anything which will be a scientific approach to the subject.

What is the use of such knowledge? In the first place, knowledge itself is the highest reward of knowledge, and secondly, there is also utility in it. It will take away all our misery. When by analysing his own mind, man comes face to face, as it were, with something which is never destroyed, something which is, by its own nature, eternally pure and perfect, he will no more be miserable, no more unhappy. All misery comes from fear, from unsatisfied desire.

Man will find that he never dies, and then he will have no more fear of death. When he knows that he is perfect, he will have no more vain desires, and both these causes being absent, there will be no more misery—there will be perfect bliss, even while in this body.

There is only one method by which to attain this knowledge, that which is called concentration. The chemist in his laboratory concentrates all the energies of his mind into one focus and throws them upon the materials he is analysing, and so finds out their secrets. The astronomer concentrates all the energies of his mind and projects them through his telescope upon the skies, and the stars, the sun, and the moon give up their secrets to him. The more I can concentrate my thoughts on the matter on which I am telling you, the more light I can throw upon you. You are listening to me, and the more you concentrate your thoughts, the more clearly you will grasp what I have to say.

How has all the knowledge in the world been gained but by the concentration of the powers of the mind? The world is ready to give up its secrets if we only know how to knock, how to give it the necessary blow. The strength and force of the blow come through concentration. There is no limit to the power of the human mind. The more concentrated it is, the more power is brought to bear on one point; that is the secret.

It is easier to concentrate the mind on external things, the mind naturally goes outwards; but not so in the case of religion, or psychology, or metaphysics, where the subject and the object are one. The object is internal, the mind itself is the object, and it is necessary to study the mind itself—mind studying mind. We know that there is the power of the mind called reflection. I am talking to you. At the same time I am standing aside, as it were, a second person, and knowing and hearing what I am talking. You work and think at the same time, while a portion of your mind stands by and sees what you are thinking.

The powers of the mind should be concentrated and turned back upon itself, and as the darkest places reveal their secrets before the penetrating rays of the sun, so will this concentrated mind penetrate its own innermost secrets. Thus will we come to the basis of belief, the real genuine religion. We will perceive for ourselves whether we have souls, whether life is of five minutes, or of eternity, whether there is a God in the universe or none. It will all be revealed to us.

This is what Rajayoga proposes to teach. The goal of all its teachings is how to concentrate the mind, then, how to discover the innermost recesses of our own minds, then, how to generalise their contents and form our own conclusions from them. It, therefore, never asks the question what our religion is, whether we are Deists, or Atheists, whether Christians, Jews, or Buddhists. We are human beings; that is sufficient. Every human being has the right and the power to seek for religion. Every human being has the right to ask the reason why, and to have his question answered by himself, if he only takes the trouble.

So far, then, we see that in the study of the Rajayoga no faith or belief is necessary. Believe nothing until you find it out for yourself; that is what it teaches us. Truth requires no prop to make it stand. Do you mean to say that the facts of our awakened state require any dreams or imagings to prove them? Certainly not.

This study of Rajayoga takes a long time and constant practice. A part of this practice is physical, but mainly it is mental. As we proceed we shall find how intimately the mind is connected with the body. If we believe that the mind is simply a finer part of the body, and that mind acts upon the body, then it stands to reason that the body must react upon the mind. If the body is sick, the mind becomes sick also. If the body is healthy, the mind remains healthy and strong. When one is angry, the mind becomes disturbed. Similarly, when the mind is disturbed, the body also becomes disturbed. With the majority of mankind the mind is greatly under the control of the body, their mind being very little developed.

The vast mass of humanity is very little removed from the animals. Not only so, but in many instances, the power of control in them is little higher than that of the lower animals. We have very little command of our minds. Therefore, to bring that command about, to get that control over body and mind, we must take certain physical helps. When the body is sufficiently controlled, we can attempt the manipulation of the mind. By manipulating the mind, we shall be able to bring it under our control, make it work as we like, and compel it to concentrate its powers as we desire.

According to the Rajayogi, the external world is but the

gross form of the internal or subtle. The finer is always the cause, the grosser the effect. So the external world is the effect, the internal the cause. In the same way, external forces are simply the grosser parts, of which the internal forces are the finer. The man who has discovered and learnt how to manipulate the internal forces will get the whole of nature under his control.

The yogi proposes to himself no less a task than to master the whole universe, to control the whole of nature. He wants to arrive at the point where what we call "nature's laws" will have no influence over him, where he will be able to get beyond them all. He will be master of the whole of nature, internal and external. The progress and civilisation of the human race simply mean controlling this nature.

Different races take to different processess of controlling nature. Just as in the same society some individuals want to control the external nature, and others the internal, so, among races, some want to control the external nature, and others the internal. Some say that by controlling the internal nature we control everything. Others say that by controlling the external nature we control everything.

Carried to the extreme both are right because in nature there is no such division as internal or external. These are fictitious limitations that never existed. The externalists and the internalists are destined to meet at the same point, when both reach the extreme of their knowledge. Just as a physicist, when he pushes his knowledge to its limits, finds it melting away into metaphysics, so a metaphysician will find that what he calls mind and matter are but apparent distinctions, the reality being One.

The end and aim of all science is to find the unity, the One out of which the manifold is being manufactured, that One existing as many. Rajayoga proposes to start from the internal world, to study the internal nature, and, through that, control the whole—both internal and external. It is a very old attempt. India has been its special stronghold, but it was also attempted by other nations. In Western countries it was regarded as mysticism and people who wanted to practise it were either burned or killed as witches and sorcerers. In India, for various reasons, it fell into the hands of persons who destroyed ninety per cent of the knowledge, and tried to make a great secret of the remainder. In modern times many so-called teachers have arisen in the West worse than those of India, because the latter knew something while these modern exponents knew nothing.

Anything that is secret and mysterious in these systems of yoga should be at once rejected. The best in life is strength. In religion, as in all other matters, discard everything that weakens you, have nothing to do with it. Mystery-mongering weakens the human brain. It has well-nigh destroyed yoga—one of the grandest of sciences. **From the time it was discovered, more than four thousand years ago, yoga was perfectly delineated, formulated, and preached in India.**

It is a striking fact that the more modern the commentator, the greater the mistakes he makes, while the more ancient the writer, the more rational he is. Most of the modern writers talk of all sorts of mystery. Thus yoga fell into the hands of a few persons who made it a secret, instead of letting the full blaze of daylight and reason fall upon it. They did so that they might have the powers to themselves.

In the first place there is no mystery in what I teach. What little I know I will tell you. So far as I can reason it out I will do so, but as to what I do not know I will simply tell you what the books say. It is wrong to believe blindly. You must exercise your own reason and judgment; you must practise and see whether these things happen or not. Just as you would take up any other science, exactly in the same manner you should take up this science for study. There is neither mystery nor danger in it. So far as it is true, it ought to be preached in the public streets in broad daylight. Any attempt to mystify these things is productive of great danger.

Before proceeding further, I will tell you a little of the Sankhya philosophy, upon which the whole of Rajayoga is based. According to the Sankhya philosophy, the genesis of perception is as follows: the affections of external objects are carried by the outer instruments to their respective brain centres or organs, the organs carry the affections to the mind, the mind to the determinative faculty, from this the Purusha (the soul) receives them, when perception results. Next he gives the order back, as it were, to the motor centres to do the needful. With the exception of the Purusha all of these are material, but the mind is much finer matter than the external instruments.

That material of which the mind is composed goes also to form the subtle matter called the *Tanmatras*. These become gross and make the external matter. That is the psychology of the Sankhya. So that between the intellect and the grosser matter outside there is only a difference in degree. The Purusha is the only thing which is immaterial. The mind is an instrument, as it were, in the hands of the soul, through which the soul catches external objects. The mind is constantly changing and vacillating, and can, when perfected, either attach itself to several organs, to one, or to none.

For instance, if I hear the clock with great attention, I will not, perhaps, see anything although my eyes may be open, showing that the mind was not attached to the seeing organ, while it was to the hearing organ. But the perfected mind can be attached to all the organs simultaneously. It has the reflexive power of looking back into its own depths.

This reflexive power is what the yogi wants to attain; by concentrating the powers of the mind, and turning them inward he seeks to know what is happening inside. There is in this no question of mere belief; it is the analysis arrived at by certain philosophers.

Modern physiologists tell us that the eyes are not the organ of vision, but that the organ is in one of nerve centres of the brain, and so with all the senses; they also tell us that these centres are formed of the same material as the brain itself. The Sankhya also tells us the same thing. The former is a statement on the physical side, and the latter on the psychological side; yet both are the same. Our field of research lies beyond this.

The yogi proposes to attain that fine state of perception in which he can perceive all the different mental states. There must be mental perception of all of them. One can perceive how the sensation is travelling, how the mind is receiving it, how it is going to the determinative faculty, and how this gives it to the Purusha. As each science requires certain preparations and has its own method, which must be followed before it could be understood, even so in Rajayoga.

Certain regulations as to food are necessary; we must use that food which brings us the purest mind. If you go into a menagerie, you will find this demonstrated at once. You see the elephants, huge animals, but calm and gentle; and if you go towards the cages of the lions and tigers, you find them restless, showing how much difference has been made by food. All the forces that are working in this body have been produced out of food; we see that every day. If you begin to fast, first your body will get weak, the physical forces will suffer; then after a few days, the mental forces will suffer also. First, memory will fail. Then comes a point, when you are not able to think, much less to pursue any course of reasoning.

We have, therefore, to take care what sort of food we eat at the begining and when we have got strength enough, when our practice is well advanced, we need not be so careful in this respect. While the plant is growing, it must be hedged round, lest it be injured; but when it becomes a tree, the hedges are taken away. It is strong enough to withstand all assaults.

A yogi must avoid the two extremes of luxury and austerity. He must not fast, nor torture his flesh. He who does so, says the Gita, cannot be a yogi: "He who fasts, he who keeps awake, he who sleeps much, he who works too much, he who does no work, none of these can be a yogi." (Gita, VI. 16)

2

The First Steps

Rajayoga is divided into eight steps. The first is **Yama**—non-killing, truthfulness, non-stealing, continence, and non-receiving of any gifts. Next is **Niyama**—cleanliness, contentment, austerity, study, and self-surrender to God. Then comes **Asana**, or posture; **Pranayama**, or control of Prana; **Pratyahara** or restraint of the senses from their objects; **Dharana** or fixing the mind on a stop; **Dhyana,** or meditation; and **Samadhi,** or super consciousness.

The Yama and Niyama, as we see, are moral trainings; without these as the basis no practice of yoga will succeed. As these two become established, the yogi will begin to realise the fruits of his practice; without these it will never bear fruit. A yogi must not think of injuring anyone, by thought, word, or deed. Mercy shall not be for men alone, but shall go beyond, and embrace the whole world.

The next step is Asana, posture. A series of exercises, physical and mental, is to be gone through every day, untill certain higher states are reached. Therefore, it is quite necessary that we should find a posture in which we can remain long. That posture which is the easiest for one should be the one chosen. For thinking, a certain posture may be very easy for one man, while to another it may be very difficult.

We will find later on that during the study of these psychological matters a good deal of activity goes on in the body. Nerve currents will have to be displaced and given a new channel. New sorts of vibrations will begin, the whole constitution will be remodelled, as it were. But the main part of the activity will lie along the spinal column, so that the one thing necessary for the posture is to hold the spinal column free, sitting erect, holding the three parts--the chest, neck, and head--in a straight line.

Let the whole weight of the body be supported by the ribs, and then you have an easy natural posture, with the spine straight. You will easily see that you cannot think very high thoughts with the chest in. This portion of the yoga is a little similar to the Hathayoga which deals entirely with the physical body, its aim being to make the physical body very strong. We have nothing to do with it here, because its practices are very difficult, and cannot be learnt in a day, and, after all, do not lead to much spiritual growth. Many of these practices you will find in some teachers, such as placing the body in diffierent postures, but the object in these is physical, not psychological. There is not one muscle in the body over which a man cannot establish perfect control. The heart can be made to stop or go on at his bidding, and each part of the organism can be similarly controlled.

The result of this branch of yoga is to make men live long; health is the chief idea, the one goal of the Hathayogi. He is determined not to fall sick, and he never does. He lives long; a hundred years is nothing to him. He is quite young and fresh when he is 150, without one hair turned grey. But that is all. A banyan tree lives sometimes 5000 years, but it is a banyan tree and nothing more. So, if a man lives long, he is only a healthy animal.

One or two ordinary lessons of the Hathayogis are very useful. For instance, some of you will find it a good thing for headaches to drink cold water through the nose as soon as you get up in the morning; the whole day your brain will be nice and cool, and you will never catch cold. It is very easy to do; put your nose into the water, draw it up through the nostrils and make a pump action in the throat.

After one has learnt to have a firm erect seat, one has to perform, according to certain schools, a practice called the purifying of the nerves. This part has been rejected by some as not belonging to Rajayoga, but as so great an authority as the commentator Shankaracharya advises it, thinks fit that it should be mentioned, and I will quote his own directions from his commentary on the Shvetashvatara Upanishad:

> The mind whose dross has been cleared away by Pranayama becomes fixed in Brahman; therefore Pranayama is declared. First the nerves are to be purified, then comes the power to practise Pranayama. Stopping the right nostril with the thumb, through the left nostril fill in air, according to capacity; then, without any interval, throw the air out through the right nostril, closing the left one. Again inhaling through the right nostril eject through the left, according to capacity; practising this three or five times at four hours of the day, before dawn, during midday, in the evening, and at midnight; in fifteen days or a month purity of the nerves is attained; then begins Pranayama.

Practice is absolutely necessary. You may sit down and read it by the hour every day, but if you do not practise, you will not get one step further. It all depends on practice. We never understand these things until we experience them. We will have to see and feel them for ourselves. Simply listening to explanations and theories will not do.

There are several obstructions to practice. The first obstruction is an unhealthy body; if the body is not in a fit state, the practice will be obstructed. Therefore, we have to keep the body in good health; we have to take care what we eat and drink, and what we do. Always use a mental effort to keep the body strong. That is all—nothing further of the body. We must not forget that health is only a means to an end. If health were the end, we would be like animals; animals rarely become unhealthy.

The second obstruction is doubt; we always feel doubtful about things we do not see. Man cannot live upon words, however he may try. So doubt comes to us as to whether there is any truth in these things or not; even the best of us will doubt sometimes. With practice, within a few days, a little glimpse will come, enough to give one encouragement and hope. As a certain commentator on yoga philosophy says, "When one proof is obtained, however little that may be, it will give us faith in the whole teaching of yoga."

For instance, after the first few months of practice, you will begin to find you can read another's thoughts; they will come to you in picture form. Perhaps you will hear something happening at a long distance, when you concentrate your mind with a wish to hear. These glimpses will come, by little bits at first, but enough to give you faith, and strength, and hope. For instance, if you concentrate your thoughts on the tip of your nose, in a few days you will begin to smell most beautiful fragrance, which will be enough to show you that there are certain mental perceptions that can be made obvious without the contact of physical objects.

But we must always remember that these are only the means; the aim, the end, the goal of all this training is liberation of the soul. Absolute control of nature, and nothing short of it, must be the goal. We must be the masters, and not the slaves of nature; neither body nor mind must be our master, nor must we forget that the body is mine, and not I the body's.

A god and a demon went to learn about the Self from a

great sage. They studied with him for a long time. At last the sage told them, "You yourself are the Being you are seeking." Both of them thought that their bodies were the Self. They went back to their people quite satisfied and said, "We have learnt everything that was to be learnt; eat, drink, and be merry; we are the Self; there is nothing beyond us." The nature of the demon was ignorant, clouded, so he never inquired any further, but was perfectly contented with the idea that he was God, that by the Self was meant the body.

The god had a purer nature. He at first committed the mistake of thinking, "I, this body, am Brahman; so keep it strong and in health, and well dressed, and give it all sorts of enjoyments." But, in a few days, he found out that that could not be the meaning of the sage, their master; there must be something higher. So he came back and said, "Sir, did you teach me that this body was the Self? If so, I see all bodies die; the Self cannot die." The sage said, "Find it out; thou art That." Then the god thought that the vital forces which work the body were what the sage meant.

But, after a time, he found that if he ate, these vital forces remained strong, but, if he starved, they became weak. The god then went back to the sage and said, "Sir, do you mean that the vital forces are the Self?" The sage said, "Find out for yourself; thou art That." The god returned home once more, thinking that it was the mind, perhaps, that was the Self, but in a short while he saw that thoughts were so various, now good, again bad; the mind was too changeable to be the Self.

He went back to the sage and said, "Sir, I do not think that the mind is the Self; did you mean that?"

"No," replied the sage, "thou art That, find out for yourself."

The god went home, and at last found that he was the Self, beyond all thought, One, without birth or death, whom the sword cannot pierce or the fire burn, whom the air cannot dry or the water melt, the beginningless and endless, the immovable, the intangible, the omniscient, the omnipotent Being; that it was neither the body nor the mind, but beyond them all. So he was satisfied; but the poor demon did not get the truth, owing to his fondness for the body.

This world has a good many of these demoniac natures, but there are some gods too. If one proposes to teach any science to increase the power of sense-enjoyment, one find multitudes ready for it. If one undertakes to show the supreme goal, one finds few to listen to him. Very few have the power to grasp the higher, fewer still the patience to attain to it. But there are a few also who know that even if the body can be made to live for a thousand years, the result in the end will be the same.

When the forces that hold it together go away, the body must fall. No man was ever born who could stop his body one moment from changing. Body is the name of a series of changes. "As in a river the masses of water are changing before you every moment, and new masses are coming, yet taking similar form, so is it with this body." Yet the body must be kept strong and healthy. It is the best instrument we have.

This human body is the greatest body in the universe, and a human being the greatest being. Man is higher than all animals, than all angels; none is greater than man. Even the Devas (gods) will have to come down again and attain to salvation through a human body. Man alone attains to perfection, not even the Devas.

According to the Jews and Mohammedans, God created man after creating the angels and everything else, and after creating man. He asked the angels to come and salute him, and all did so except Iblis; so God cursed him and he became Satan. Behind this allegory is the great truth that this human birth is the greatest birth we can have. The lower creation, the animal, is dull, and manufactured mostly out of Tamas. Animals cannot have any high thoughts, nor can the angels, or Devas, attain to direct freedom without human birth.

In human society, in the same way, too much wealth or too much poverty is a great impediment to the higher development of the soul. It is from the middle classes that the great ones of the world come. Here the forces are very equally adjusted and balanced.

Returning to our subject, we come next to Pranayama, controlling the breathing. What has that to do with concentrating the powers of the mind? **Breath is like the fly-wheel of this machine, the body. In a big engine you find the fly-wheel first moving, and that motion is conveyed to finer and finer machinery until the most delicate and finest mechanism in the machine is in motion.** The breath is that fly-wheel supplying and regulating the motive power to everything in this body.

There was once a minister to a great king. He fell into disgrace. The king, as a punishment, ordered him to be shut up in the top of a very high tower. This was done, and the minister was left there to perish. He had a faithful wife, however, who came to the tower at night and called to her husband at the top to know what she could do to help him. He told her to return to the tower the following night and bring with her a long rope, some stout twine, pack thread, silken thread, a beetle, and a little honey. Wondering much, the good wife obeyed her husband, and brought him the desired articles. The husband directed her to attach the silken thread firmly to the beetle, then to smear its horns with a drop of honey, and to set it free on the wall of the tower, with its head pointing upwards.

She obeyed all these instructions, and the beetle started on its long journey. Smelling the honey ahead it slowly crept onwards, in the hope of reaching the honey, until at last it reached the top of the tower, when the minister grasped the beetle, and got possession of the silken thread. He told his wife to tie the other end to the pack thread, and after he had drawn up the pack thread, he repeated the process with the stout twine and lastly with the rope. Then the rest was easy. The minister descended from the tower by means of the rope, and made his escape.

In this body of ours the breath motion is the "silken thread"; by laying hold of it and of the nerve currents, and from these the stout twin of our thoughts, and lastly the rope of prana, controlling which we reach freedom.

We do not know anything about our own bodies, we cannot know. At best we can take a dead body and cut it into pieces, and there are some who can take a live animal and cut it into pieces in order to see what is inside the body. Still, that has nothing to do with our own bodies. We know very little about them. Why do we not? Because our attention is not discriminating enough to catch the very fine movements that are going on within.

We can know of them only when the mind becomes more subtle and enters, as it were, deeper into the body. To get the subtle perceptions we have to begin with the grosser perceptions. We have to get hold of that which is setting the whole engine in motion. That is the Prana, the most obvious manifestation of which is the breath. Then, along with the breath, we shall slowly enter the body, which will enable us to find out about the subtle forces, the nerve currents that are moving all over the body.

As soon as we perceive and learn to feel them, we shall begin to get control over them, and over the body. The mind is also set in motion by these different nerve currents, so at last we shall reach the state of perfect control over the body and the mind, making both our servants. Knowledge is power. We have to get this power. So we must begin at the beginning, with Pranayama, restraining the Prana. This Pranayama is a long subject, and will take several lessons to illustrate it thoroughly. We shall take it part by part.

We shall gradually see the reasons for each exercise and what forces in the body are set in motion. All these things will come to us, but it requires constant practice, and the proof will come by practice. No amount of reasoning which I can give you will be proof to you, until you have demonstrated it for yourselves. As soon as you begin to feel these currents in motion all over you, doubts will vanish, but it requires hard pratice every day. You must practise at least twice every day, and the best times are towards the morning and the evening. When night passes into day, and day into night, a state of relative calmness ensues.

The early morning and the early evening are the two periods of calmness. Your body will have a like tendency to become calm at those times. We should take advantage of that natural condition and begin then to practise. Make it a rule not to eat until you have practised; if you do this, the sheer force of hunger will break your laziness. In India they teach children never to eat until they have practised or worshipped, and it becomes natural to them after a time; a boy will not feel hungry untill he has bathed and practised.

Those of you who can afford it will do better to have a room for this practice alone. Do not sleep in that room, it must be kept holy. You must not enter the room until you have bathed, and are perfectly clean in body and mind. Place flowers in that room always; they are the best surroundings for a yogi; also pictures that are pleasing. Burn incense morning and evening. Have no quarrelling, nor anger, nor unholy thoughts in that room. Only allow those persons to enter it who are of the same thought as you. Then gradually there will be an atmosphere of holiness in the room, so that when you are miserable, sorrowful, or your mind is disturbed, the very fact of entering that room will make you calm.

This was the idea of the temple and the church, and in some temples and churches you will find it even now, but in a majority of them the very idea has been lost. The idea is that by keeping holy vibrations there the place becomes and remains illumined. Those who cannot afford to have a room set apart can practise anywhere they like. Sit in a straight posture, and the first thing to do is to send a current of holy thought to all creation. Mentally repeat, "Let all things be happy; let all beings be peaceful; let all beings be blissful." So do to the East, South, North, and West.

The more you do that, the better you will feel for yourself. You will find at last that the easiest way to make ourselves healthy is to see that others are healthy, and the easiest way to make ourselves happy is to see that others are happy. After doing that, those who believe in God should pray -- not for money, not for health, nor for heaven; pray for knowledge and light; every other prayer is selfish. Then the next thing to do is to think of your own body, and see that it is strong and healthy; it is the best instrument you have. Think of it as being as strong and adamant, and that with the help of this body you will cross the ocean of life. Freedom is never to be reached by the weak. Throw away all weakness. Tell your body that it is strong, tell your mind it is strong, and have unbounded faith and hope in yourself.

3

Prana is Central

Pranayama is not, as many think, something about breath; breath indeed has very little to do with it, if anything. Breathing is only one of the many exercises through which we get to the real Pranayama. Pranayama means the control of Prana.

According to the philosophers of India, the whole world is composed of two materials, one of which they call *Akasha*. It is the Omnipresent, all-penetrating existence. Everything that has form, everyting that is the result of combination, is evolved out of this Akasha. It is the Akasha that becomes the air, that becomes the liquids, that becomes the solids; it is the Akasha that becomes the sun, the earth, the moon, the stars, the comets; it is the Akasha that becomes the human body, the animal body, the plants, every form that we see, everything that can be sensed, everything that exists.

It cannot be perceived; it is so subtle that it is beyond all ordinary perception; it can only be seen when it has become gross, has taken form. At the beginning of creation there is only this Akasha. At the end of the cycle the solids, the liquids, and the gases all melt into the Akasha again, and the next creation similarly proceeds out of this Akasha.

By what power is this Akasha manufactured into this universe? By the power of Prana. Just as Akasha is the infinite, omnipresent material of this universe, so is this Prana the infinite, omnipresent manifesting power of this universe. At the beginning and at the end of a cycle everything becomes Akasha, and all the forces that are in the universe resolve back into the Prana; in the next cycle, out of this Prana is evolved everything that we call energy, everything that we call force.

It is the Prana that is manifesting as motion; it is the Prana that is manifesting as gravitation, as magnetism. It is the Prana that is manifesting as the actions of the body, as the nerve currents, as thought force. From thought down to the lowest force, everything is but the manifesting of Prana. The sum total of all forces in the lowest force, everything is but the manifestation of Prana. The sum total of all forces in the universe, mental or physical, when resolved back to their original state, is called Prana.

"When there was neither aught nor naught, when darkness was covering darknes, what existed then? That Akasha existed without motion." The physical motion of the Prana was stopped, but it existed all the same. At the end of a cycle the energies now displayed in the universe quiet down and become potential. At the begining of the next cycle they start up, strike upon the Akasha, and out of the Akasha evolve these various forms, and as the Akasha changes, this Prana changes also into all these manifestations of energy. The knowledge and control of this Prana is really what is meant by Pranayama.

This opens to us the door to almost unlimited power. Suppose, for instance, a man understood the Prana perfectly, and could control it, what power on earth would not be his? He would be able to move the sun and stars out of their places, to control everything in the universe, from the atoms to the biggest suns, because he would control the Prana. This is the end and aim of Pranayama.

When the yogi becomes perfect, there will be nothing in nature not under his control. If he orders the gods or the souls of the departed to come, they will come at his bidding, All the forces of nature will obey him as slaves. When the ignorant see these powers of the yogi, they call them the miracles. One peculiarity of the Hindu mind is that it always inquires for the last possible generalisation, leaving the details to be worked out afterwards. The question is raised in the Vedas, "What is that, knowing which, we shall know everything?"

Thus, all books, and all philosophies that have been written, have been only to prove that power by knowing which everything is known. If a man wants to know this universe bit by bit he must know every individual grain of sand, which means infinite time, yet he cannot know all of them.

Then how can knowledge be? How is it possible for a man to be all-knowing through particulars? The yogis say that behind this particular manifestation there is a generalisation. Behind all particular ideas stands a generalised, an abstract principle; grasp it, and you have grasped everything. Just as this whole universe has been generalised, in the Vedas, into that One Absolute Existence, and he who has grasped that Existence, grasped the whole universe, so all forces have been generalised into this Prana, and he who has grasped the Prana has grasped all the forces of the universe, mental or physical.

He who has controlled the Prana has controlled his own mind, and all the minds that exist. He who has controlled the Prana has controlled his body and all the bodies that exist, because the Prana is the generalised manifestation of force.

How to control the Prana is the one idea of Pranayama. All the trainings and exercises in this regard are for that one end. Each man must begin where he stands, must learn how to control the things that are nearest to him. This body is very near to us, nearer than anything in the external universe, and this mind is the nearest of all. The Prana which is working this mind and body is the nearest to us of all the Prana in the universe. This little wave of the Prana which represents our own energies, mental and physical, is the nearest to us of all the waves of the infinite ocean of Prana. If we can succeed in controlling that little wave, then alone we can hope to control the whole of Prana.

The yogi who has done this gains perfection; no longer is he under any power. He becomes almost almighty, almost all-knowing. We see sects in every country who have attempted this control of Prana. In America there are mind-healers, faith-healers, spiritualists, Christian Scientists, hypnotists, etc., and if we examine these different bodies, we shall find at the back of each this control of the Prana, whether they know it or not. If you boil all their theories down, the residuum will be that. It is the one and the same force they are manipulating, only unknowingly. They have stumbled on the discovery of a force and are using it uconsciously without knowing its nature, but it is the same as the yogi uses, and which comes from Prana.

The Prana is the vital force in every being. **Thought is the finest and highest action of Prana. Thought, again, as we see, is not all. There is also what we call instinct or unconscious thought, the lowest plane of action.** If a mosquito stings us, our hand will strike it automatically, instinctively. This is one experssion of thought. All reflex actions of the body belong to this plane of thought.

There is again the other plane of thought, the conscious. I reason, I judge, I think, I see the pros and cons of certain things, yet that is not all. We know that reason is limited. Reason can go only to a certain extent, beyond that it cannot reach. The circle within which it runs is very very limited indeed. Yet at the same time, we find facts rush into this circle. Like the coming of comets certain things come into this circle; it is certain they come from outside the limit, although our reason cannot go beyond. The causes of the phenomena intruding themselves in this small limit are outside of this limit.

The mind can exist on a still higher plane, the superconscious. When the mind has attained to the state which is called Samadhi--perfect concentration, superconciousness--it goes beyond the limits of reason, and comes face to face with facts which no instinct or reason can ever know. All manipulations of the subtle forces of the body, the different manifestations of Prana, if trained, give a push to the mind, help it to go up higher, and become superconscious, from where it acts.

In this universe there is one continuous substance on every plane of existence. Physically this universe is one; there is no difference between the sun and you. The scientist will tell you it is only a fiction to say the contrary. There is no real difference between the table and me; the table is one point in the mass of matter, and I another point. Each form represents, as it were, one whirlpool in the infinite ocean of matter, of which not one is constant.

Just as in a rushing stream there may be millions of whirlpools, the water in each of which is different every moment, turning round and round for a few seconds, and then passing out, replaced by a fresh quantity, so the whole universe is one constantly changing mass of matter, in which all forms of existence are so many whirlpools, A mass of matter enters into one whirlpool, say, a human body, stays there for a period, becomes changed, and goes out into another, say, an animal body this time, from which again after a few years, it enters into another whirlpool, called a lump of mineral.

It is a constant change. Not one body is constant. There is no such thing as my body, or your body, except in words. Of the one huge mass of matter, one point is called a moon, another a sun, another a man, another the earth, another a plant, another a mineral. Not one is constant, but everything is changing, matter eternally concreting and disintegrating. So it is with the mind. Matter is represented by the ether: when the action of Prana is most subtle, this very ether, in the finer state of vibration, will represent the mind, and there it will be still one unbroken mass.

If you can simply get to that subtle vibration, you will see and feel that the whole universe is composed of subtle vibrations. Sometimes certain drugs have the power to take us, while as yet in the senses, to that condition. Many of you may remember the celebrated experiment of Humphrey Davy, when the laughing gas overpowered him—how, during the lecture, he remained motionless, stupefied and, after he said that the whole universe was made up of ideas. For the time being, as it were, the gross vibrations had ceased, and only the subtle vibrations which he called ideas, were present to him. He could only see the subtle vibrations round him; everything had become thought; the whole universe was an ocean of thought, he and everyone else had become little thought whirlpools.

Thus, even in the universe of thought we find unity, and as last, when we get to the Self, we know that that Self can only be One. Beyond the vibrations of matter in its gross and subtle aspects, beyond motion there is but One. Even in manifested motion there is only unity. These facts can no more be denied. Modern physics also has demonstrated that the sum total of the energies in the universe is the same throughout. It has also been proved that this sum total of energy exists in two forms. It becomes potential, toned down, and calmed, and next it comes out manifested as all these various forces; again it goes back to the quiet state, and again it manifests. Thus it goes on evolving and involving through eternity. The control of this Prana, as stated, before is what is called Pranayama.

The most obvious manifestation of this Prana in the

human body is the motion of the lungs. If that stops, as a rule, all the other manifestations of force in the body will immediately stop. But there are persons who can train themselves in such a manner that the body will live on, even when this motion has stopped. There are some persons who can bury themselves for days, and yet live without breathing. To reach the subtle we must take the help of the grosser, and so, slowly travel towards the most subtle until we gain our point.

Pranayama really means controlling this motion of the lungs, and this motion is associated with the breath. Not that breath is producing it; on the contrary, it is producing breath. This motion draws in the air by pump action. **The Prana is moving the lungs, the movement of the lungs draws in the air. So Pranayama is not breathing, but controlling that muscular power which moves the lungs.** That muscular power which goes out through the nerves to the muscles and from them to the lungs, making them move in a certain manner, is the Prana, which we have to control in the practices of Pranayama. When the Prana has become controlled, then we shall immediately find that all the other actions of the Prana in the body will slowly come under control.

I myself have seen men who have controlled almost every muscle of the body; and why not? If I have control over certain muscles, why not over every muscle and nerve of the body? What impossibility is there? At present the control is lost, and the motion has become automatic. We cannot move our ears at will, but we know that animals can. We have not that power because we do not exercise it. This is what is called atavism.

Again, we know that motion which has become latent can be brought back to manifestation. By hard work and practice certain motions of the body which are most dormant can be brought back under perfect control.

Reasoning thus we find there is no impossibility, but, on the other hand, every probability that each part of the body can be brought under perfect control. This the yogi does through Pranayama. Perhaps some of you have read that in Pranayama, when drawing in the breath, you must fill your whole body with Prana. In the English translations Prana is given as Breath, and you are inclined to ask how that is to be done. The fault is with the translator. Every part of the body can be filled with Prana, this vital force, and when you are able to do that, you can control the whole body. All the sickness and misery felt in the body will be perfectly controlled; not only so you will be able to control another's body.

Everything is infectious in this world, good or bad. If your body be in a certain state of tension, it will have a tendency to produce the same tension in others. If you are strong and healthy, those who love near you will also have the tendency to become strong and healthy but if you are sick and weak, those around you will have the tendency to become the same. In the case of one man trying to heal another, the first idea is simply transferring his own health to the other. This is the primitive sort of healing.

Consciously or unconsciously, health can be transmitted. A very strong man, living with a weak man, will make him a little stronger, whether he knows it or not. When consciously done, it becomes quicker and better in its action. Next come those cases in which a man may not be very healty himself, yet we know that he can bring health to another. The first man, in such a case, has a little more control over the Prana, and can arouse, for the time being, his Prana, as it were, to a certain state of vibration, and transmit it to another person.

There have been cases where this process has been carried on at a distance, but in reality there is no distance in the sense of a break. Where is the distance that has a break? Is there any break between you and the sun? It is a continuous mass of matter. Is there a break between one part of a river and another? Then why cannot any force travel? There is no reason against it. Cases of healing from a distance are perfectly true. The Prana can be transmitted to a very great distance; but to one genuine case, there are hundreds of frauds.

This process of healing is not so easy as it is thought to be. In the most ordinary cases of such healing you will find that the healers simply take advantage of the naturally healthy state of the human body. An allopath comes and treats cholera patients, and gives them his medicines. The homoeopath comes and gives his medicines and cures perhaps more than the allopath does, because the homoeopath does not disturb his patients, but allows nature of deal with them. The faith-healer cures more still, because he brings the strength of his mind to bear, and rouse through faith the dormant Prana of the patient.

There is a mistake constantly made by faith-healers: they think that faith directly heals a man. But faith alone does not cover all the ground. There are diseases where the worst symptoms are that the patient never thinks that he has that disease. That tremendous faith of the patient is itself one symptom of the disease, and usually indicates that he will die quickly. In such cases the principle that faith cures does not apply. If it were faith alone that cured, these patients also would be cured.

It is by the Prana, that real curing comes. **The pure man, who has controlled the Prana, has the power of bringing it into a certain state of vibrations, which can be conveyed to others arousing in them a similar vibration.** You see that in every day actions. I am talking to you. What am I trying to do? I am, so to say, bringing my mind to a certain state of vibration, and the more I succeed in bringing it to that state, the more you will be affected by what I say. All of you know that the day I am more enthusiastic, the more you enjoy the lecture; and when I am less enthusiastic, you feel lack of interest.

The gigantic will-powers of the world, the world-movers, can bring their Prana into a high state of vibration, and it is so great and powerful that it catches others in a moment, and thousands are drawn towards them, and half the world thinks as they do. Great prophets of the world had the most wonderful control of the Prana, which gave them tremendous will-power; they had brought their Prana to the highest state of motion and this is what gave them the power to sway the world.

All manifestations of power arise from this control. Men may not know the secret, but this is the one explanation. Sometimes in your own body the supply of Prana gravitates more or less to one part; the balance is disturbed, what we call disease is produced. To take away the superfluous Prana, or to supply the prana that is wanting, will be curing the disease. That again is Pranayama—to learn when there is more or less Prana in one part of the body than there should be. The feelings will become so subtle that the mind will feel that there is less Prana in the toe or the finger than there should be, and will possess the power to supply it.

These are among the various functions of Pranayama. They have to be learnt slowly and gradually, and as you see, the whole scope of Raja-yoga is really to teach the control and direction in different planes of the Prana. When a man has concentrated his energies, he masters the Prana that is in his body. When a man is meditating, he is also concentrating the Prana.

In an ocean there are huge waves, like mountains, then smaller waves, and still smaller, down to little bubbles, but back of all these is the infinite ocean. The bubble is connected with the infinite ocean at one end, and the huge wave at the other end. So, one may be a gigantic man, and another a little bubble, but each is connected with that infinite ocean of energy, which is the common birthright of every animal that exists.

Wherever there is life, the storehouse of infinite energy is behind it. Starting as some fungus, some very minute, microscopic bubble, and all the time drawing from that infinite storehouse of energy, a form is changed slowly and steadily, until in course of time it becomes a plant, then an animal, then a man, ultimately God. This is attained through millions of aeons, but what is Time? An increase of speed, an increase of struggle, is able to bridge the gulf of Time. That which naturally takes a long time to accomplish can be shortened by the intensity of the action, says the yogi.

A man may go on slowly drawing in this energy from the infinite mass that exists in the universe, and, perhaps, he will require a hundred thousand year to become a Deva, and then perhaps, five hundred thousand years to become still higher, and perhaps, five millions of years to become perfect. Given rapid growth, the time will be lessened. Why is it not possible, with suffcient effort, to reach this very perfection in six months or six years?

There is no limit. Reason shows that. If an engine, with a certain amount of coal, runs two miles an hour, it will run the distance in less time with a greater supply of coal. Similarly, why shall not soul, by intensifying its action, attain perfection in this very life? All beings will at last attain to that goal, we know. But who cares to wait all these millions of aeons? Why not reach it immediately, in this body even, in this human form? Why shall I not get that infinite knowledge, infinite power, now?

The ideal of the yogi, the whole science of yoga, is directed to the end of teaching men how, by intensifying the power of assimilation, to shorten the time for reaching perfections, instead of slowly advancing from point to point and waiting until the whole human race has become perfect. All the great prophets, saints, and seers of the world—what did they do? In one span of life they lived the whole length of time that it takes ordinary humanity to come to perfection. In one life they perfect themselves; they have no thought for anything else, never live a moment for any other idea, and thus the way is shortened for them. This is what is meant by concentration, intensifying the power of assimilation, thus shortening the time. Rajayoga is the science which teaches us how to gain the power of concentration.

What has Pranayama to do with spiritualism? Spiritualism is also a manifestation of Pranayama. if it be true that the departed spirits exist, only we cannot see them, it is quite probable that there may be hundreds and millions of them about us we can neither see, feel, nor touch. We may be continually passing and repassing through their bodies, and they do not see or feel us. It is a circle within a circle, universe within universe.

We have five senses, and we represent Prana in a certain state of vibration. All beings in the same state of vibration will see one another but if there are beings who represent Prana in a higher state of vibration, they will not be seen. We may increase the intensity of a light until we cannot see it all, but there may be beings with eyes so powerful that they can see such light. Again, if its vibrations are very low, we do not see a light, but there are animals that may see it, as cats and owls.

Our range of vision is only one plane of the vibrations of this Prana. Take this atmosphere, for instance; it is piled up layer on layer, but the layers nearer to the earth are denser than those above, and as you go higher the atmosphere becomes finer and finer. Or take the case of the ocean; as you go deeper and deeper the pressure of the water increases and animals which live at the bottom of the sea can never come up, or they will be broken into pieces.

Think of the universe as an ocean of ether, consisting of layer after layer of varying degrees of vibration under the action of Prana; away from the centre the vibrations are less, nearer to it they become quicker and quicker; one order of vibration makes one plane. Then suppose these ranges of vibrations are cut into planes, so many millions of miles one set of vibrations and then so many millions of miles another still higher set of vibrations, and so on.

It is, therefore, probable, that those who live on the plane of a certain state of vibration will have the power of recognising one another, but will not recognise those above them. Yet, just as by the telescope and the microscope we can increase the scope of our vision, similarly, we can by yoga bring ourselves to the state of vibration of another plane, and thus enable ourselves to see what is going on there. Suppose this room is full of beings whom we do not see. They represent Prana in a certain state of vibration while we represent another. Suppose they represent a quick one, and we the opposite.

Prana is the material of which they are composed, as well as we. All are parts of the same ocean of Prana, they differ only in their rate of vibration. If I can bring myself to the quick vibration, this plane will immediately change for me: I shall not see you any more; you vanish and they appear. Some of you, perhaps, know this to be true.

All this bringing of the mind into a higher state of vibrations is included in one word in yoga—Samadhi. All these states of higher vibrations, superconscious vibrations of the mind, are grouped in that one word, Samadhi, and the lower states of Samadhi give us visions of these beings. The highest grade of Samadhi is when we see the real things, when we see the material out of which the whole of these grades of beings are composed, and the one lump of clay being known, we know all the clay in the universe.

Thus we see that Pranayama includes all that is true of spiritualism even. Similarly, you will find that wherever any sect or body of people is trying to search out anything occult and mystical, or hidden, what they are doing is really this yoga, this attempt to control the Prana. You will find that wherever there is any extraordinary display of power, it is the manifestation of this Prana.

Even the physical sciences can be included in Pranayama. What moves the steam engine? Prana, acting through the steam. What are all these phenomena of electricity and so forth but Prana! What is physical science? The science of Pranayama, by external means. Prana, manifesting itself as mental power, can only be controlled by mental means. That part of Pranayama which attempts to control the physical manifestations of the Prana by physical means is called physical science, and that part which tries to control the manifestations of the Prana as mental force, by mental means, is called Rajayoga.

4

The Psychic Prana

According to the yogis, there are two nerve currents in the spinal column, called Pingala and Ida, and a hollow canal called Sushumnã running through the spinal cord. At the lower end of the hollow canal is what the yogis call the "Lotus of the Kundalini." They desribe it as triangular in form, in which in the symbolical language of the yogis, there is a power called the Kundalini, coiled up. **When the Kundalini awakes, it tries to force a passage through this hollow canal, and as it rises step by step, as it were, layer after layer of the mind becomes open and all the different visions and wonderful powers come to the yogi.** When it reaches the brain, the yogi is perfectly detached from the body and mind; the soul finds itself free.

We know that the spinal cord is composed in a peculiar manner. If we take the figure eight horizontally (∞) there are two parts which are connected in the middle. Suppose you add eight after eight, piled one on top of the other, that will represent the spinal cord. The left is the Ida, the right Pingala, and that hollow canal which runs through the centre of the spinal cord is the Sushumna. Where the spinal cord ends in some of the lumbar vertebrae, a fine fibre issues downwards, and the canal runs up even within that fibre, only much finer. The canal is closed at the lower end, which is situated near what is called the sacral plexus, which, according to modern physiology, is triangular in form. The different plexuses that have their centres in the spinal canal can very well stand for the different "lotuses" of the yogi.

The yogi conceives of several centres, beginning with the Muladhara the basic, and ending with the Sahasrãra, the thousand-petalled lotus in the brain. So, if we take these different plexuses as representing these lotuses, the idea of the yogi can be very easily understood in the language of modern physiology. We know there are two sorts of actions in these nerve currents, one afferent, the other defferent; one sensory and the other motor; one centripetal, and the other centrifugal. One carries the sensations to the brain, and the other from the brain to the outer body. These vibrations are all connected with the brain in the long run.

Several other facts we have to remember, in order to clear the way for the explanation which is to come. The spinal cord, at the brain, ends in a sort of bulb, in the medulla, which is not attached to the brain, but floats in a fluid in the brain, so that if there be a blow on the head the force of the blow will be dissipated in the fluid, and will not hurt the bulb. This is an important fact to remember. Secondly, we have also to know that, of all the centres, we have particularly to remember three, the Muladhara (the basic), the Sahasrara (the thousand-petalled lotus of the brain) and the Manipura (the lotus of the navel).

Next we shall take one fact from physics. We all hear of electricity and various other forces connected with it. What electricity is no one knows, but so far as it is known, it is a sort of motion. There are various other motions in the universe; what is the difference between them and electricity? Suppose this moves—that the molecules which compose this table are moving in different directions; if they are all made to move in the same direction, it will be through electricity. Electric motion makes the molecules of a body move in the same direction. If all the air molecules in a room are made to move in the same direction, it will make a gigantic battery of electricity of the room.

Another point from physiology we must remember, that the centre which regulates the respiratory system, the breathing system, has a sort of controlling action over the system of nerve currents.

Now we shall see why breathing is practised. In the first place, from rhythmical breathing comes a tendency of all the molecules in the body to move in the same direction.When mind changes into will, the nerve currents change into a motion similar to electricity, because the nerves have been proved to show polarity under the action of electric currents. This shows that **when the will is transformed into the nerve currents, it is changed into something like electricity. When all the motions of the body have become perfectly rhythmical, the body has, as it were, become a gigantic battery of will.**

This tremendous will is exactly what the yogi wants. This is, therefore, a physiological explanation of the breathing exercise. It tends to bring a rhythmic action in the body, and helps us, through the respiratory centre, to control the other centres. The aim of Pranayama here is to rouse the coiled-up power in the Muladhara, called the Kundalini.

Everything that we see, or imagine, or dream, we have to perceive in space. This is the ordinary space, called the Mahakasha,or elemental space. **When a yogi reads the thoughts of other men, or perceives super-sensuous objects, he sees them in another sort of space called the Chittakasha, the mental space.** When perception has become objectless, and the soul shines in its own nature, it is called the Chidakasha, or knowledge space. When the Kundalini is aroused, and enters the canal of the Sushumna, all the perceptions are in the mental space, **when it has reached that end of the canal which opens out into the brain, the objectless perception is in the knowledge space.** Taking the analogy of electricity, we find that man can send a current only along a wire, but nature requires no wires to send her tremendous currents. This proves that the wire is not really necessary, but that only our inability to dispense with it compels us to use it.

Similarly, all the sensations and motions of the body are being sent into the brain, and sent out of it, through these wires of nerve fibres. The columns of sensory and motor fibres in the spinal cord are the Ida and Pingala of the yogis. They are the main channels through which the afferent and efferent currents travel. But why should not the mind send news without any wire, or react without any wire?

We see this is done in nature. The yogi says, if you can do that, you have got rid of the bondage of matter. How to do it? If you can make the current pass through the Sushumna, the canal in the middle of the spinal column, you have solved the problem.The mind has made this network of the nervous system, and has to break it, so that no wires will be required to work through. Then alone will all knowledge come to us—no more bondage of body, that is why it is so important that we should get control of that Sushumna. If we can send the mental current through the hollow canal without any nerve fibres to act as wires, the yogi says, the problem is solved, and he also says it can be done.

This Sushumna is in ordinary persons closed up at the lower extremity; no action comes through it. **The yogi proposes a practice by which it can be opened, and the nerve currents made to travel through.** When a sensation is carried to a centre, the centre reacts. This reaction, in the case of automatic centres, is following by motion; in the case of conscious centres it is followed first by perception, and secondly by motion.

All perception is the reaction to action from outside. How, then, do perception in dreams arise? There is then no action from outside. The sensory motions, therefore, are coiled up somewhere. For instance, I see a city; the perception ot that city is from the reaction to the sensations brought from outside objects comprising that city. That is to say, a certain motion in the brain molecules has been set up by the motion in the incarrying nerves, which again are set in motion by external objects in the city.

Now, even after a long time, I can remember the city. This memory is exactly the same phenomenon, only it is in a milder form. But whence is the action that sets up even the milder form of similar vibrations in the brain? Not certainly from the primary sensations. Therefore it must be that the sensations are coiled up somewhere, and they, by their acting, bring out the mild reaction which we call dream perception.

Now the centre where all these residual sensations are, as it were, stored up, is called the Muladhara, the root receptacle, and the coiled up energy of action is Kundalini, "the coiled up." It is very probable that the residual motor energy is also stored up in the same centre, as, after deep study of meditation on external objects, the part of the body where the Muladhara centre is situated (probably the sacral plexus) gets heated. Now, if this coiled-up energy be roused and made active, and then consciously made to travel up the Sushumna canal, as it acts upon centre after centre, a tremendous reaction will set in.

When a minute portion of energy travels along a nerve fibre and causes reaction from centres, the perception is either dream or imagination. **But when by the power of long internal meditation, the vast mass of energy stored up travels along the Sushumna, and strikes the centres, the reaction is tremendous, immensely superior to the reaction of dream or imagination,** immensely more intense than the reaction of sense-perception. It is supersensuous perception. And when it reaches the metropolis of all sensations, the brain, the whole brain, as it were, reacts, and the result is full blaze of illumination, the perception of the Self.

As this Kundalini force travels from centre to center, layer after layer of the mind, as it were, opens up, and this universe is perceived by the yogi in its fine, or causal form. Then alone the causes of this universe, both as sensation and reaction, are known as they are, and hence comes all knowledge. The causes known, the knowledge of the effects is sure to follow.

Thus, the rousing of the Kundalini is the one and only way to attaining Divine Wisdom, superconscious perception, realisation of the spirit. **The rousing may come in various ways, through love for God, through the mercy of perfected sages, or through the power of the analytic will of the philosopher.** Wherever there was any manifestation of what is ordinarily called supernatural power or wisdom, there a little current of Kundalini must have found its way into the Sushumna. Only, in the vast majority of such cases, people had ignorantly stumbled on some practice which set free a minute portion of the coiled-up Kundalini. All worship, consciously or unconsciously, leads to this end.

The man who thinks that he is receiving response to his prayers does not know that the fulfilment comes from his own nature, that he has succeeded by the mental attitude of prayer in waking up a bit of this infinite power which is coiled up within himself. What, thus, men ignorantly worship under various names, through fear and tribulation, the yogi declares to the world to be the real power coiled up in every being, the mother of eternal happiness, if we but know how to approach her. And Rajayoga is the science of religion, the rationale of all worship, all prayers, forms, ceremonies, and miracles.

5

The Control of Psychic Prana

We have now to deal with the exercises in Pranayama. We have seen that the first step, according to the yogis, is to control the motion of the lungs. What we want to do is to feel the finer motions that are going on in the body. Our minds have become externalised, and have lost sight of the fine motions inside. If we can begin to feel them, we can begin to control them. These nerve currents go on all over the body, bringing life and vitality to every muscle, but we do not feel them. The yogi says we can learn to do so. How? By taking up and controlling the motion of the lungs; when we have done that for a suffcient length of time, we shall be able to control the finer motions.

We now come to the exercises in Pranayama. Sit upright; the body must be kept straight. The spinal cord, althought not attached to the vertebral column, is yet inside of it. If you sit crookedly you disturb this spinal cord, so let it be free. **Any time that you sit crookedly and try to meditate you do yourself an injury.** The three parts of the body, the chest, the neck, and the head must be always held straight in one line.

You will find that by a little practice this will come to you as easy as breathing. The second thing is to get control of the nerves. We have said that the nerve centre that controls the respiratory organs has a sort of controlling effect on the other nerves, and rhythmical breathing is, therefore, necessary. The breathing that we generally use should not be called breathing at all. It is very irregular. Then there are some natural differences of breathing between men and women.

The first lesson is just to breathe in a measured way, in and out. That will harmonise the system. When you have practised this for some time, you will do well to join to it the repetition of some word as "Om," or any other sacred word. In India we use certain symbolical words instead of counting one, two, three, four. That is why I advise you to join the mental repetition of the "Om," or some other sacred word to the Pranayama. Let the word flow in and out with the breath, rhythmically, harmoniously, and you will find the whole body is becoming rhythmical. Then you will learn what rest is. Compared with it, sleep is not rest. Once this rest comes the most tired nerves will be calmed down, and you will find that you have never before really rested.

The first effect of this practice is perceived in the change of expression of one's face; harsh lines disappear, with calm thought calmness comes over the face. Next comes beautiful voice. I never saw a yogi with a croaking voice. These signs come after a few months' practice.

After practising the above-mentioned breathing for a few days, you should take up a higher one. Slowly fill the lungs with breath through the Ida, the left nostril, and at the same time concentrate the mind on the nerve current. You are, as it were, sending the nerve current down the spinal column, and striking violently on the last plexus, the basic lotus which is triangular in form, the seat of the Kundalini. Then hold the current there for some time.

Imagine that you are slowly drawing that nerve current with the breath through the other side, the Pingala, then slowly throw it out through the right nostril. This you will find a little difficult to practise. The easiest way is to stop the right nostril with the thumb, and then slowly draw in the breath through the left; then close both nostrils with thumb and forefinger, and imagine that you are sending that current down and striking the base of the Sushumna; then take the thumb off, and let the breath out through the right nostril.

Next, inhale slowly through that nostril, keeping the other closed by the forefinger, then close both, as before. It will be well to begin with four seconds, and slowly increase. Draw in four seconds, hold in sixteen seconds, then throw out in eight seconds. This makes one Pranayama.

At the same time think of the basic lotus, triangular in form; concentrate the mind on that centre. The imagination can help you a great deal. The next breathing is slowly drawing the breath in, and then immediately throwing it out slowly, and then stopping the breath out, using the same numbers. The only difference is that in the first case the breath was held in, and in the second, held out.

This last is the easier one. The breathing in which you hold the breath in the lungs must not be practised too much. Do it only four times in the morning, and four times in the evening. Then you can slowly increase the time and number. You will find that you take pleasure in it. So very carefully and cautiouly increase as you feel that you have the power, to six instead of four. It may injure you if you practise it irregularly.

Of the three processes for the purification of the nerves, described above, the first and the last are neither difficult nor dangerous. The more you practise the first one, the calmer you will be. Just think of 'Om' and you can practise even while you are sitting at your work. You will be all the better for it. Some day, if you practise hard the Kundalini will be aroused. For those who practise once or twice a day, just a little calmness of the body and mind will come, and beautiful voice; only for those who can go on further with it will Kundalini be aroused, and the whole of nature will begin to change and the book of knowledge will open.

No more will you need to go to books for knowledge; your own mind will have become your book, containing infinite knowledge. I have already of the Ida and Pingala currents, flowing through either side of the spinal column, and also of the Sushumna, the passage through the centre of the spinal cord. These three are present in every animal; whatever being has a spinal column has these three lines of action. But the Yogis claim that in an ordinary man the Sushumna is closed; its action is not evident while that of the other two is carrying power to different parts of the body.

The Yogi alone has the Sushumna open. When this Sushumna current opens, and begins to rise, we get beyond the senses, our minds become supersensuous, superconscious—we get beyond even the intellect, where reasoning can not reach. **To open that Sushumna is the prime object of the Yogi. According to him, along this Sushumna are ranged these centres, or, in more figurative language, these lotuses, as they are called.** The lowest one is at the lower end of the spinal cord, and is called Muladhara, the next higher is called Svadhisthana, the third Manipura, the fourth Anahata, the fifth Vishuddha, the sixth Ajna and the last, which is in the brain, is the Sahasrara, or "the thousand-petalled."

Of these we have to take cognition just now of two centres only, the lowest, the Muladhara, and the highest, the Sahasrara. All energy has to be taken up from its seat in the Muladhara and brought to the Sahasrara. The yogis claim that of all the energies that are in the human body the highest is what they call "Ojas." Now this Ojas is stored up in the brain, and the more Ojas is in a man's head, the more spiritually strong he is. One man may not speak beautiful language nor beautiful thoughts, yet his words charm. Every movement of his is powerful. That is the power of Ojas.

Now in every man there is more or less of this Ojas stored up. All the forces that are working in the body in their highest become Ojas. You must remember that it is only a question of transformation. The same force which is working outside as electricity or magnetism will become changed into inner force; the same force that is working as muscular energy will be changed into Ojas.

The yogis say that the part of **the human energy which is expressed as sex energy, in sexual thought, when checked and controlled, easily becomes changed into Ojas,** and as the Muladhara guides these, the yogi pays particular attention to that centre. He tries to take up all this sexual energy and convert it into Ojas. **It is only the chaste man or woman who can make the Ojas rise and store it in the brain; that is why chastity has always been considered the highest virtue.** A man feels that if he is unchaste, spirituality goes away, he loses mental vigour and moral stamina.

That is why in all the religious orders in the world which have produced spiritual giants you will always find absolute chastity insisted upon. That is why the monks came into existence, giving up marriage. There must be perfect chastity in thought, word, and deed; without it the practice of Rajayoga is dangerous, and may lead to insanity.

6

Pratyahara and Dharana

The next step is called Pratyahara. What is this? you know how perceptions come. First of all there are the external instruments, then the internal organs, acting in the body through the brain centres, and there is the mind. When these come together and attach themselves to some external object, then we perceive it. At the same time it is a very difficult thing to concentrate the mind and attach it to one organ only; the mind is a slave.

We hear "Be good," "Be good," and "Be good" is taught all over the world. There is hardly a child, born in any country in the world, who has not been told, "Do not steal." "Do not tell a lie," but nobody tells the child how he can help doing them. Talking will not help him. Why should he not become a thief? We do not teach him how not to steal, we simply tell him, "Do not steal," Only when we teach him to control his mind do we really help him.

All actions, internal and external, occur when the mind joins itself to certain centres, called the organs. Willingly or unwillingly it is drawn to join to the centres, and that is why people do foolish deeds and feel miserable, which, if the mind were under control, they would not do. What would be the result of controlling the mind? It then would not join itself to the centres of perception, and, naturally, feeling and willing would be under control. It is clear so far.

Is it possible? It is perfectly possible. You see it in modern times; the faith-healers teach people to deny misery and pain and evil. Their philosophy is rather roundabout, but it is a part of yoga upon which they have somehow stumbled. Where they succeed in making a person throw off suffering by denying it, they really use a part of Pratyahara, as they make the mind of the person strong enough to ignore the senses. The hypnotists in a similar manner, by their suggestion, excite in the patient a sort of morbid Pratyahara for the time being. The so-called hypnotic suggestion can only act upon a weak mind. And until the operator, by means of fixed gaze or otherwise, has succeeded in putting the mind of the subject in a sort of passive, morbid condition, his suggestions never work.

Now the control of the centres which is established in a hypnotic patient or the patient of faith-healing by the operator, for the time, is reprehensible, because it leads to ultimate ruin. It is not really controlling the brain centres by the power of one's own will, but is, as it were, stunning the patient's mind for a time by sudden blows which another's will delivers to it. It is not checking by means of reins and muscular strength the mad career of a fiery team, but rather by asking another to deliver heavy blows on the heads of the horses to stun them for a time into gentleness. At each one of these processes the man operated upon loses a part of his mental energies, till at last, the mind, instead of gaining the power of perfect control, becomes a shapeless, powerless mass, and the only goal of the patient is the lunatic asylum.

Every attempt at control which is not voluntary, not with the controller's own mind, is not only disastrous, but it defeats the end. The goal of each soul is freedom, mastery—freedom from the slavery of matter and thought, mastery of external and internal nature. Instead of leading towards that, every will-current from another, in whatever form it comes, either as direct control of organs, or as forcing to control them while under a morbid condition, only heavy chain of bondage of past thoughts, past superstitions.

Therefore, beware how you allow yourselves to be acted upon by others. Beware how you unknowingly bring another to ruin. True, some succeed in doing good to many for a time, by giving a new trend to their propensities, but at the same time, they bring ruin to millions by the unconscious suggestions they throw around, rousing in men and women that morbid, passive hypnotic conditions which makes them almost soulless at last. Whosoever, therefore, asks anyone to believe blindly, or drags people behind him by the controlling power of his superior will, does an injury to humanity, though he may not intend it.

Therefore, use your own minds, control body and mind yourselves, remember that until you are a diseased person, no extraneous will can work upon you; avoid everyone, however great and good he may be, who asks you to believe blindly. All over the world there have been dancing and jumping and howling sects, who spread like infection when they begin to sing and dance and preach; they also are a sort of hypnotists. They exercise a singular control for the time being over sensitive persons, alas! often, in the long run, to degenerate whole races. It is healthier for the individual or the race to remain wicked than be made apparently good by such morbid extraneous control.

One's heart sinks to think of the amount of injury done to humanity by such irreponsible, yet well-meaning religious fanatics. They little know that the minds which attain to sudden spiritual upheaval under their suggestions, with music and prayers, are simply making themselves passive, morbid, and powerless, and opening themselves to any other suggestion, be it ever so evil. Little do these ignorant, deluded persons dream that, whilst they are congratulating themselves upon their miraculous power to transform human hearts, which power they think was poured upon them by some Being above the clouds, they are sowing the seeds of future decay, of crime, of lunacy, and of death. Therefore, beware of everything that takes away your freedom. Know that it is dangerous, and avoid it by all the means in your power.

He who has succeeded in attaching or detaching his mind to or from the centres at will has succeeded in Pratyahara, which means, "gathering towards," checking the outgoing powers of the mind, freeing it from the thraldom of the senses. When we can do this, we shall really possess character; then alone we shall have taken a long step towards freedom; before that we are mere machines.

How hard it is to control the mind! Well has it been compared to the maddened monkey. There was a monkey, restless by his own nature, as all monkeys are. As if that were not enough, some one made him drink freely of wine, so that he become still more restless. Then a scorpion stung him. When a man is stung by a scorpion he jumps about for a whole day; so the poor monkey found his condition worse than ever. To complete his misery a demon entered into him. What language can describe the uncontrollable restlessness of that monkey?

The human mind is like that monkey, incessantly active by its own nature; then it becomes drunk with the wine of desire, thus increasing its turbulence. After desire takes possession comes the sting of the scorpion of jealousy at the success of others, and last of all the demon of pride enters the mind, making it think itself of all importance. How hard to control such a mind!

The first lesson, then is to sit for some time and let the mind run on. The mind is bubbling up all the time. It is like that monkey jumping about. Let the monkey jump as much as he can; you simply wait and watch. Knowledge is power, says the proverb, and that is true. Until you know what the mind is doing you cannot control it. Give if the rein; many hideous thoughts may come into it; you will be astonished that it was possible for you to think such thoughts. But you will find that each day the mind's vagaries are becoming calmer.

In the first few months you will find that the mind will have a great many thoughts, later you will find that they have somewhat decreased, and in a few more months they will be fewer and fewer, until at last the mind will be under perfect control, but we must patiently practise every day. As soon as the steam is turned on, the engine must run; as soon as things are before us we must perceive; so a man, to prove that he is not a machine, must demonstrate that he is under the control of nothing. This controlling of the mind, and not allowing it to join itself to the centres is Pratyahara. How is this practised? It is tremendous work, not to be done in a day. Only after a patient, continuous struggle for years can we succeed .

After you have practised Pratyahara for a time, take the next step, the Dharana holding the mind to certain points. What is meant by holding the mind to certain points? Forcing the mind to feel certain parts of the body to the exclusion of others. For instance, try to feel only the hand, to the exclusion of other parts of the body. **When the Chitta, or mind-stuff is confined and limited to a certain place, it is Dharana.** This Dharana is of various sorts, and along with it, it is better to have a little play of the imagination. For instance, the mind should be made to think of one point in the heart. That is very difficult; an easier way is to imagine a lotus there. That lotus is full of light, effulgent light. Put the mind there. Or think of the lotus in the brain as full of light, or of the different centres in the Sushumna mentioned before.

The yogi must always practise. He should try to live alone; the companionship of different sorts of people distracts the mind; he should not speak much, because to speak distracts the mind; not work much, because too much work distracts the mind; the mind cannot be controlled after a whole day's hard work. One observing the above rules becomes a yogi. Such is the power of yoga that even the least of it will bring a great amount of benefit. It will not hurt anyone, but will benefit everyone.

First of all, it will tone down nervous excitement, bring calmness, enable us to see things more clearly. The temperament will be better, and the health will be better. Sound health will be one of the first signs, and a beautiful voice. Defects in the voice will be changed. This will be among the first of the many effects that will come. Those who practise hard will get many other signs. Sometimes there will be sounds, as a peal of bells heard at a distance, commingling and falling on the ear as one continuous sound. Sometimes things will be seen, little specks of light floating and becoming bigger and bigger; and when these things come, know that you are progressing fast.

Those who want to be yogis, and practice hard, must take care of their diet at first. But for those who want only a little practice for everyday business sort of life, let them not eat too much; otherwise they may eat whatever they please. For those who want to make rapid progress, and to practise hard, a strict diet is absolutely necessary. They will find it advantageous to live only on milk and cereals for some months. As the organisation becomes finer and finer, it will be found in the beginning that the least irregularity throws one out of balance. One bit of food more or less will disturb the whole system, until one gets perfect control, and then one will be able to eat whatever one likes.

When one begins to concentrate, the dropping of a pin will seem like a thunderbolt going through the brain. As the organs get finer, the perceptions get finer. These are the stages through which we have to pass, and all those who persevere will succeed. Give up all argumentation and other distractions. Is there anything in dry intellectual jargon? It only throws the mind off its balance and disturbs it. Things of subtler planes have to be realised. Will talking do that? So give up all vain talk. Read only those books which have been written by persons who have had realisation.

Be like the pearl oyster. There is a pretty Indian fable to the effect that if it rains when the star Svati is in the ascendant, and a drop of rain falls into an oyster, that drop becomes a pearl. The oysters know this, so they come to the surface when that star shines, and wait to catch the precious raindrop. When a drop falls into them, quikly the oysters close their shells and dive down to the bottom of the sea, there to patiently develop the drop into the pearl. We should be like that.

First, hear, then understand, and then, leaving all distractions, shut your minds to outside influences, and devote yourselves to developing the truth within you. There is the danger of frittering away your energies by taking up an idea only for its novelty, and then giving it up for another that is newer. Take one thing up and do it, and see the end of it, and before you have seen the end, do not give it up. He who can become mad with an idea, he alone sees light. Those that only take a nibble here and a nibble there will never attain anything. They may titillate their nerves for a moment, but there it will end. They will be slaves in the hands of Nature, and will never get beyond the senses.

Those who really want to be yogis must give up, once for all, this nibbling at things. Take up one idea. Make that one idea your life--think of it, dream of it, live on that idea. Let the brain, muscles, nerves, every part of your body, be full of that idea, and just leave everuy other idea alone. This is the way to success, and this is the way great spiritual giants are produced. Others are mere talking machines. If we really want to be blessed, and make others blessed, we must go deeper.

The first step is not to disturb the mind, not to associate with persons whose ideas are disturbing. All of you know that certain persons, certain places, certain foods, repel you. Avoid them; and those who want to go to the highest, must avoid all company, good or bad. Practise hard; whether you live or die does not matter. You have to plunge in and work, without thinking of the result. If you are brave enough, in six months you will be a perfect yogi. But those who take up just a bit of it and a little of everything else make no progress.

It is of no use simply to take a course of lessons. To those who are full of Tamas, ignorant and dull--those whose minds never get fixed on any idea, who only crave for something to amuse them—religion and philosophy are simply objects of entertainment. These are the unpersevering. They hear a talk, think it very nice, and then go home and forget all about it. To succeed, you must have tremendous perseverance, tremendous will. "I will drink the ocean," says the persevering soul, "at my will mountains will crumble up." Have that sort of energy, that sort of will, work hard, and you will reach the goal.

7

Dhyana and Samadhi

We have taken a cursory view of the different step in Rajayoga, except the finer ones, the training in concentration, which is the goal, to which Rajayoga will lead us. We see, as human beings, that all our knowledge which is called rational is referred to consciousness. My consciousness of this table, and of your presence, makes me know that the table and you are here. At the same time, there is a very great part of my existence of which I am not conscious. All the different organs inside the body, the different parts of the brain—nobody is conscious of these.

When I eat food, I do it consciously; when I assimilate it, I do it unconsiously. When the food is manufactured into blood, it is done unconsciously. When out of the blood all the different parts of my body are strengthened, it is done unconsciously. And yet it is I who am doing all this; there cannot be twenty people in this one body. How do I know that I do it, and nobody else? It may be urged that my business is only in eating and assimilating the food, and that strengthening the body by the food is done for me by somebody else. That cannot be, because it can be demonstrated that almost every action of which we are now unconscious, can be brought up to the plane of consciousness.

The heart is beating apparently without our control. None of us here can control the heart; it goes on its own way. But by practice men can bring even the heart under control, until it will just beat at will, slowly, or quickly, or almost stop. Nearly every part of the body can be brought under control. What does this show? That the functions which are beneath consciousness are also performed by us, only we are doing it unconsciously. We have, then, two planes in which the human mind works.

First is the conscious plane, in which all work is always accompanied with the feeling of egoism. Next comes the unconscious plane, where all work is unaccompanied by the feeling of egoism. That part of mind-work which is unaccompanied with the feeling of egoism is conscious work. In the lower animals this unconscious work is called instinct. In higher animals, and in the highest of all animals, man, what is called conscious work prevails.

But it does not end here. There is a still higher plane upon which the mind can work. It can go beyond consciousness. Just as unconscious work is beneath consciousness, so there is another work which is above consciousness and which also is not accompanied with the feeling of egoism. **The feeling of egoism is only on the middle plane. When the mind is above or below that line, there is no feeling of "I", and yet the mind works. When the mind goes beyond this line of self-consciousness, it is called Samadhi, or super-consciousness.**

How, for instance, do we know that a man in samadhi has not gone below consciousness, has not degenerated instead of going higher? In both cases the works are unaccompanied with egoism. The answer is, by the effects, by the results of the work,we know that which is below, and that which is above. When a man goes into deep sleep, he enters a plan beneath consciousness. He works the body all the time, he breathes, he moves the body, perhaps, in his sleep, without any accompanying feeling of ego; he is unconscious, and when he returns from his sleep, he is the same man who went into it. The sum total of the knowledge which he had before he went into the sleep remains the same; it does not increase at all. No enlightenment comes. But when a man goes into samadhi, if he goes into it a fool, he comes out a sage.

What makes the difference? From one state a man comes out the very same that he went in, and from another state the man comes out enlightened, a sage, a prophet, a saint, his whole character changed, his life changed, illumined. These are the two effects. Now the effects being different the causes must be different. As this illumination with which a man comes back from samadhi is much higher than can be got from unconsciousness, or much higher than can be got by reasoning in a conscious state, it must, therefore, be super-consciousness, and samadhi is called the super-conscious state.

This, in short, is the idea of samadhi. What is its application? The application is here. The field of reason, or of the conscious working of the mind, is narrow and limited. There is a little circle within which human reason must move. It cannot go beyond. Every attempt to go beyond is impossible, yet it is beyond this circle of reason that there lies all the humanity holds most dear. All these questions, whether there is an immortal soul, whether there is a God, whether there is any supreme intelligence guiding this universe or not, are beyond the field of reason. Reason can never answer these questions.

What does reason say? It says, "I am agnostic; I do not know either yea or nay." Yet these questions are so important to us. Without a proper answer to them, human life will be purposeless. All our ethical theories, all our moral attitudes, all that is good and great is human nature, have been moulded upon answers that have come from beyond the circle. It is very important, therefore, that we should have answers to these question. If life is only a short play, if the universe is only a short play, if the universe is only a "fortuitious combination of atoms," then why should I do good to another? Why should there by mercy, justice, or fellow-feeling? The best thing for this world would be to make hay while the sun shines, each man for himself.

If there is no hope, why should I love my brother, and not cut his throat? If there is nothing beyond, if there is no feedom, but only rigorous dead laws, I should only try to make myself happy here. You will find people saying that they have utilitarian ground as the basis of morality. What is this basis? Procuring the greatest amount of happiness to the greatest number. Why should I do this? Why should I not produce the greatest unhappiness to the greatest number, if that serves my purpose?

How will utilitarians answer this question? How do you know what is right, or what is wrong? I am impelled by my desire for happiness, and I fulfil it, and it is in my nature; I know nothing beyond. I have these desires, and must fulfil them, why should you complain? Whence come all these truths about human life, about morality, about the immortal soul, about God, about love and sympathy, about being good, and, above all, about being unselfish?

All ethics, all human action, and all human throught, hang upon this one idea of unselfishness. The whole idea of human life can be put into that one word, unselfishness. Why should we be unselfish? Where is the necessity, the force, the power, of my being unselfish? You call yourself a rational man, a utilitarain; but if you do not show me a reason for utility, I say you are irrational. Show me the reason why I should not be selfish? To ask one to be unselfish may be good as poetry, but poetry is not reason. Show me a reason. Why shall I be unselfish, and why be good? Because Mr. and Mrs. So-and-so say so does not weigh with me. Where is the utillity of my being unselfish? My utility means the greatest amount of happiness.

What is the answer? The utilitarian can never give it.

The answer is that this world is only one drop in an infinite ocean, one link in an infinite chain. Where did those that preached unselfishness, and taught it to the human race, get this idea? We know it is not instinctive; the animals, which have insinct, do not know it. Neither is it reason, reason does not know anything about these ideas. Whence then did they come?

We find, in studying history, one fact held in common by all the great teachers of religion the world ever had. They all claim to have got their truths from beyond, only many of them did not know where they got them from. For instance, one would say that an angel came down in the form of a human being, with wings, and said to him, "Hear, O man, this is the message." Another says that a Deva, a bright being, appeared to him. A third says he dreamed that his ancestor came and told him certain things. He did not know anything beyond that. But this is common that all claim that this knowledge has come to them from beyond, not through their reasoning power.

What does the science of yoga teach? It teaches that they were right in claiming that all this knowledge came to them from beyond reasoning, but that it came from within themselves.

The yogi teaches that the mind itself has a higher state of existence, beyond reason, a superconscious state, and when the mind gets to that higher state, then this knowledge, beyond reasoning, comes to man. Metaphysical and transcendental knowledge comes to that man. This state of going beyond reason, transcending ordinary human nature, may sometimes come by chance to a man who does not understand its science; he as it were, stumbles upon it. When he stumbles upon it, he generally interprets it as coming from outside.

So this explains why an inspiration, or transcendental knowledge, may be the same in different countries, but in one country it will seem to come through an angel, and in another through a Deva, and in a third through God. What does it mean? It means that the mind brought the knowledge by its own nature, and that the finding of the knowledge was interpreted according to the belief and education of the person through whom it came. The real fact is that these various men as it were, stumbled upon this superconscious state.

The yogi says there is a great danger in stumbling upon this state. In a good many cases there is the danger of the brain being deranged, and, as a rule, you will find that all those men, however great they were, who had stumbled upon this super-conscious state without understanding it, groped in the dark, and generally had, along with their knowledge, some quaint superstition. They opened themselves to hallucinations. Mohammed claimed that the Angel Gabriel came to him in a cave one day and took him on the heavenly horse, Harak, and he visited the heavens. But with all that, Mohammed spoke some wonderful truths. If you read the Koran, you find the most wonderful truths mixed with superstitions.

How will you explain it? That man was inspired, no doubt, but that inspiration was, as it were, stumbled upon. He was not a trained yogi, and did not know the reason of what he was doing. Think of the good Mohammed did to the world, and think of the great evil that has been done through his fanaticism! Think of the millions massacred through his teachings, mothers bereft of their children, children made orphans, whole countries destroyed, millions upon millions of people killed!

So we see this danger by studying the lives of great teachers like Mohammed and others. Yet we find, at the same time, that they were all inspired. Whenever a prophet got into the super-conscious state by heightening his emotional nature, he brought away from it not only some truths, but some fanaticism also, some superstition which injured the world as much as the greatness of the teaching helped. To get any reason out of the mass of incongruity we call human life, we have to transcend our reason, but we must do it scientifically, slowly, by regular practice, and we must cast off all superstition.

We must take up the study of the super-conscious state just as any other science. On reason we must have to lay our foundation, we must follow reason as far as it leads, and when reason fails, reason itself will show us the way to the highest plane. When you hear a man say. "I am inspired", and then talk irrationally, reject it. Why? Because these three states—instinct, reason, and super-consciousness, or the unconscious, conscious, and super-conscious states—belong to one and the same mind.

There are not three minds in one man, but one state of it develops into the others. Instinct develops into reason, and reason into the transcendental consciousness; therefore, not one of the states contradicts the others. Real inspiration never contradicts reason, but fulfils it. Just as you find the great prophets saying, "I come not to destroy but to fulfil," so inspiration always comes to fulfil reason, and is in harmony with it.

All the different steps in yoga are intended to bring us scientifically to the super-conscious state, or Samadhi. Furthermore, this is a most vital point to understand, that inspiration is as much in every man's nature as it was in that of the ancient prophets. These prophets were not unique; they were men as you or I; they were great yogis. They had gained this super-consciousness, and you and I can get the same. They were not peculiar people. The very fact that one man ever reached that state, proves that it is possible for every man to do so. Not only is it possible, but every man must, eventually, get to that state, and that is religion.

Experience is the only teacher we have. We may talk

and reason all our lives, but we shall not understand a word of truth, until we experience it ourselves. You cannot hope to make a man a surgeon by simply giving him a few books. You cannot satisfy my curiosity to see a country by showing me a map; I must have actual experience. Maps can only create curiosity in us to get more perfect knowledge. Beyond that, they have no value whatever. Clinging to books only degenerates the human mind.

Was there ever a more horrible blasphemy than the statement that all the knowledge of God is confined to this or that book? How dare men call God infinite, and yet try to compress him within the covers of a little book! Millions of people have been killed because they did not believe what the books said, because they would not see all the knowledge of God within the covers of a book. Of course, this killing and mudering has gone by, but the world is still tremendously bound up in a belief in books.

In order to reach the super-conscious state in a scientific manner it is necessary to pass through the various steps of Rajayoga. After Pratyahara and Dharana we come to Dhyana, meditation. When the mind has been trained to remain fixed on a certain internal or external location, there comes to it the power of flowing in an unbroken current, as it were, towards that point. This state is called Dhyana. When one has so intensified the power of Dhyana as to be able to reject the external part of perception and remain mediating, that state is called Samadhi.

The three—Dharana, Dhyana, and Samadhi—together are called Samyama. That is, if the mind can first concentrate upon an object, and then is able to continue in that concentration for a length of time, and then, by continued concentration, to dwell only on the internal part of the perception of which the object was the effect, everything comes under the control of such a mind.

This meditative state is the highest state of existence.

So long as there is desire, no real happiness can come. It is only the contemplative, witness-like study of objects that brings to us real enjoyment and happiness. The animal has its happiness in the senses, the man in his intellect, and the god in spiritual contemplation. It is only to the soul that has attained to this contemplative state that the world really becomes beautiful. To him who desires nothing, and does not mix himself up with them, the manifold changes of nature are one panorama of beauty and sublimity.

These ideas have to be understood in Dhyana or meditation. We hear a sound. First there is the external vibration; second, the nerve motion that carries it to the mind; third, the reaction from the mind, along with which flashes the knowledge of the object which was the external cause of these different changes from the ethereal vibrations to the mental reactions.

These three are called in yoga, Shabda (sound), Artha (meaning), and Jnana (knowledge). In the language of physics and physiology they are called the ethereal vibration, the motion in the nerve and brain, and the mental reaction. Now these, though distinct processes, have become mixed up in such a fashion as to become quite indistinct. In fact, we cannot now perceive any of these, we only perceive their combined effect, what we call the external object. Every act of perception includes these three, and there is no reason why we should not be able to distinguish them.

When, by the previous preparations, it becomes strong and controlled, and has the power of finer perception, the mind should be employed in meditation. This meditation must begin with gross objects and slowly rise to finer and finer, until it becomes objectless. The mind should first be employed in perceiving the external causes of sensations, then the internal motions, and then its own reaction. When it has succeeded in perceiving the external causes of sensations by themselves, the mind will acquire the power of perceiving all fine material existences, all fine bodies and forms.

When it can succeed in perceiving the motions inside by themselves, it will gain the control of all mental waves, in itself or in others, even before they have translated themselves into physical energy; and when he will be able to perceive the mental reaction by itself, the yogi will acquiire the knowledge of everything, as every sensible object, and every thought, is the result of this reaction. Then will he have seen the very foundations of his mind, and it will be under his perfect control. Different powers will come to the yogi, and, if he yields to the temptation of any one of these, the road to his further progress will be barred.

Such is the evil of running after enjoyments. But if he is strong enough to reject even these miraculous powers, he will attain to the goal of yoga, the complete suppression of the waves in the ocean of the mind. Then the glory of the soul, undisturbed by the distractions of the mind, or motions of the body, will shine in its full effulgence; and the yogi will find himself as he is and as he always was, the essence of knowledge, the immortal, the all-pervading.

Samadhi is the property of every human being--nay, every animal. From the lowest animal to the highest angel, some time or other, each one will have to come to that state, and then, and then alone, will real religion begin for him. Until then we only struggle towards that stage. There is no difference now between us and those who have no religion, because we have no experience. What is concentration good for, save to bring us to this experience? Each one of the steps to attain Samadhi has been reasoned out, properly adjusted, scientifically organised, and when faithfully practised, will surely lead us to the desired end. Then will all sorrows cease, all miseries vanish; the seeds for actions will be burned, and the soul will be free for ever.

II

The Classic Patanjali's YOGA SUTRA

•

Commentary by

SWAMI VIVEKANANDA

1

Spiritual Uses of Concentration

अथ योगानुशासनम् ॥1॥

Now concentration is explained.

योगश्चित्तवृत्तिनिरोधः ॥2॥

Yoga is restraining the mind-stuff (Chitta) from taking various forms (Vrittis).

A good deal of explanation is necessary here. We have to understand what Chitta is, and what the Vrittis are. I have eyes. Eyes do not see. Take away the brain centre which is in the head, the eyes will still be there, the retina complete, as also the pictures of objects on them, and yet the eyes will not see. So the eyes are only a secondary instrument, not the organ of vision. The organ of vision is in a nerve centre of the brain.

The two eyes will not be sufficient. Sometimes a man is asleep with his eyes open. The light is there and the picture is there, but a third thing is necessary—the mind must be joined to the organ. The eyes are the external instrument; we need also the brain centre and the agency of the mind.

Carriages roll down a street, and you do not hear them. Why? Because your mind has not attached itself to the organ of hearing. First, there is the instrument, then there is the organ, and third the mind attached to these two. The mind takes the impression farther in, and presents it to the determinative faculty—Buddhi—, which reacts.

Along with this reaction flashes the idea of egoism.

Then this mixture of action and reaction is presented to the Purusha, the real Soul, who perceives an object in this mixture. The organs (Indriyas), together with the mind (Manas), the determinative faculty (Buddhi), and egoism (Ahamkara), form the group called the Antahkarana (the internal instrument); they are but various processes in the mind stuff, called Chitta.

The waves of thought in the Chitta are called Vrittis (literally "whirlpool").

What is thought? Thought is a force, as is gravitation or repulsion. From the infinite storehouse of force in nature, the instrument called Chitta takes hold of some, absorbs it and sends it out as thought. Force is supplied to us through food, and out of that food the body obtains the power of motion, etc. Others, the finer forces, it throws out in what we call thought.

So we see that the mind is not intelligent; yet it appears to be intelligent. Why? Because the intelligent soul is behind it. You are the only sentient being; mind is only the instrument through which you catch the external world.

Take a book; as a book it does not exist outside, what exists outside is unknown and unknowable. The unknowable furnishes the suggestion that gives a blow to the mind, and the mind gives out the reaction in the form of a book, in the same manner as when a stone is thrown into the water, the water is thrown against it in the form of waves.

The real universe is the occasion of the reaction of the mind. A book form, or an elephant form, or a man form, is not outside; all that we know is our mental reaction from the outer suggestion. "Matter is the permanent possibility of sensations." said John Stuart Mill. It is only the suggestion that is outside.

Take an oyster for example. You know how pearls are made. A parasite gets inside the shell and causes irritation, and the oyster throws a sort of enameling round it, and this makes the pearl. The universe of experience is our own enamel, so to say, and the real universe is the parasite serving as nucleus. The ordinary man will never understand it, because when he tries to do so, he throws out an enamel, and sees only his own name.

Now we understand what is meant by these Vrittis. The real man is behind the mind; the mind is the instrument in his hands; it is his intelligence that is percolating through the mind. It is only when you stand behind the mind that it becomes intelligent. When man gives it up, it falls to pieces and is nothing. Thus you understand what is meant by Chitta. It is the mind-stuff, and Vrittis are the waves and ripples rising in it when external causes impinge on it. These Vrittis are our universe.

The bottom of a lake we cannot see, because its surface is covered with ripples. It is only possible for us to catch a glimpse of the bottom, when the ripples have subsided, and the water is calm. If the water is muddy or is agitated all the time, the bottom will not be seen. If it is clear, and there are no waves, we shall see the bottom. The bottom of the lake is our own true Self; the lake is the Chitta and the waves the Vrittis.

Again, the mind is in three states, one of which is darkness, called Tamas, found in brutes and idiots; it only acts to injure. No other idea comes into that state of mind, Then there is the active state of mind, Rajas whose chief motives are power and enjoyment. "I will be powerful and rule others." Then there is the state called Sattva, serenity, calmness, in which the waves cease, and the water of the mind-lake becomes clear. It is not inactive, but rather intensely active. It is the greatest manifestation of power to be calm. It is easy to be active. Let the reins go, and the horses will run away with you. Anyone can do that, but he who can stop the plunging horses is the strong man. Which requires the greater strength, letting go or restraining?

The calm man is not the man who is dull. You must not mistake Sattva for dullness or laziness. The calm man is the one who has control over the mind waves. Activity is the manifestation of inferior strength, and calmness of the superior.

The Chitta is always trying to get back to its natural pure state, but the organs draw it out. To restrain it, to check this outward tendency, and to start it on the return journey to the essence of intelligence, is the first step in yoga, because only in this way can the Chitta get into its proper course.

Although the Chitta is in every animal from the lowest to the highest, it is only in the human form that we find it as the intellect. Until the mind-stuff can take the form of intellect, it is not possible for it to return through all these steps, and liberate the soul. Immediate salvation is impossible for the cow or the dog, Although they have mind, because their Chitta cannot as yet take that form which we call intellect.

The Chitta manifests itself in the following form—scattering, darkening, gathering, one-pointed, and concentrated. The scattering form is activity. Its tendency is to manifest in the form of pleasure or of pain. The darkening form is dullness which tends to injury. The commentator says, the third form is natural to the devas, the angels, and the first and second to the demons. The gathering form is when it struggles to centre itself. The one-pointed form is when it tries to concentrate, and the concentrated form is what brings us to Samadhi.

तदा द्रष्टुः स्वरूपेऽवस्थानम् ॥3॥

At that time [the time of concentration] The seer [Purusha] rest in his own [unmodified] state.

As soon as the waves have stopped, and the lake has

become quiet, we see its bottom. So with the mind; when it is calm, we see what our own nature is; we do not mix ourselves but remain our own selves.

वृत्तिसारूप्यमितरत्र ॥4॥

At other times other than that of concentration] the seer is identified with the modifications.

For instance, someone blames me; this produces a modification, Vritti, in my mind, and I identify myself with it, and the result is misery.

वृत्तयः पञ्चतय्यः क्लिष्टाऽक्लिष्टाः ॥5॥

There are five classes of modifications. (some) painful and (others) not painful.

प्रमाण-विपर्यय-विकल्प-निद्रा-स्मृतयः ॥6॥

[These are] right knowledge, indiscrimi-nation, verbal delusion, sleep and memory.

प्रत्यक्षानुमानागमाः प्रमाणानि ॥7॥

Direct perception, inference and competent evidence, are proofs.

When two of our perceptions do not contradict each other, we call it proof. I hear something, and if it contradicts something already perceived, I begin to fight it out, and do not believe it.

There are also three kinds of proof. Direct perception, Pratyaksha, whatever we see, feel, is proof, if there has been nothing to delude the senses. I see the world; that is sufficient proof that it exists. Secondly, Anumana, inference; you see a sign, and from the sign you come to the thing signified. Thirdly, Aptavakya, the direct evidence of the yogis, of those who have seen the truth. We are all of us struggling towards knowledge. But you and I have to struggle hard, and come to knowledge through a long tedious process of reasoning, but the yogi, the pure one, has gone beyond all this. Before his mind, the past, the present, and the future are alike, one book for him to read; he does not require to go through the tedious processes for knowledge we have to; his words are proof, because he sees knowledge in himself.

These, for instance, are the authors of the sacred scriptures; therefore the scriptures are proof. If any such persons are living now their words will be proof. Other philosophers go into long discussions about Aptavakya and they say, "What is the proof of their words?" The proof is their direct perception. Because whatever I see is proof, and whatever you see is proof, if it does not contradict any past knowledge. There is knowledge beyond the senses, and whenever it does not contradict reason and past human experience, that knowledge is proof.

Any mad man may come into this room and say he sees angels around him; that would not be proof. In the first place, it must be true knowledge; and secondly, it must not contradict past knowledge; and thirdly, it must depend upon the character of the man who gives it out. I hear it said that the character of the man is not of so much importance as what he may say: we must first hear what he says. This may be true in other things. A man may be wicked, and yet make an astronomical discovery, but in religion it is different, because no impure man will ever have the power to reach the truths of religion.

Therefore we have first of all to see that the man who declares himself to be an Apta is a perfectly unselfish and holy person; secondly, that he has reached beyond the senses; and thirdly, that what he says does not contradict the past of humanity. Any new discovery of truth does not contradict the past truth, but fits into it. And fourthly, that truth must have a possibility of verification. If a man says, " I have seen a vision," and tells me that I have no right to see it, I believe him not. Everyone must have the power to see it for himself.

No one who sells his knowledge is an Apta. All these conditions must be fulfilled; you must first see that the man is pure, and that he has no selfish motive: that he has no thirst for gain or fame. Secondly, he must show that he is superconscious. He must give us something that we cannot get from our senses, and which is for the benefit of the world. Thirdly, we must see that it does not contradict other truths; if it contradicts other scientific truths, reject it at once. Fourthly, the man should never be singular; he should only represent what all men can attain.

The three sorts of proof are, then, direct sense perception, inference, and the words of an Apta. I cannot translate this word into English. It is not the word "inspired", because inspiration is believed to come from outside, while this knowledge comes from the man himself. The literal meaning is "attained".

विपर्ययो मिथ्याज्ञानमतद्रूपप्रतिष्ठम् ॥8॥

Indiscrimination is false knowledge not established in real nature.

The next class of Vrittis that arises is mistaking one thing for another, as a piece of mother of pearl is taken for a piece of silver.

शब्दज्ञानानुपाती वस्तुशून्यो विकल्पः ॥9॥

Verbal delusion follows from words having no (corresponding) reality.

There is another class of Vrittis called Vikalpa, A word is uttered, and we do not wait to consider its meaning; we jump to a conclusion immediately. It is the sign of weakness of the Chitta. Now you can understand the theory of restraint. The weaker the man, the less he has of restraint. Examine yourselves always by that test. When you are going to be angry or miserable, reason it out how it is that some news that has come to you is throwing your mind into Vrittis.

अभाव-प्रत्ययालम्बना वृत्तिर्निद्रा ॥10॥

Sleep is a Vritti which embraces the feeling of voidness.

The next class of Vrittis is called sleep and dream. When we awake, we know that we have been sleeping; we can only have memory of perception. That which we do not perceive we never can have any memory of. Every reaction is a wave in the lake. Now, if, during sleep, the mind had no waves, it would have no perceptions, positive or negative, and, therefore, we would not remember them.

The very reason of our remembering sleep is that during sleep there was a certain class of waves in the mind. Memory is another class of Vrittis which is called Smriti.

अनुभूतविषयासम्प्रमोषः स्मृतिः ॥11॥

Memory is when the (Vrittis of) perceived subjects do not slip away (and through impressions come back to consciousness).

Memory can come from direct perception, false knowledge, verbal delusion, and sleep. For instance, you hear a word. That word is like a stone thrown into the lake of the Chitta; it causes a ripple, and that ripple rouses a series of ripples; this is memory. So in sleep. When the peculiar kind of ripple called sleep throws the Chitta into a ripple of memory, it is called a dream. Dream is another form of the ripple which in the waking state is called memory.

अभ्यासवैराग्याभ्यां तन्निरोधः ॥12॥

Their control is by practice and non-attachment.

The mind, to have non-attachment, must be clear, good

and rational. Why should we practise? Because each action is like the pulsations quivering over the surface of the lake. The vibration dies out, and what is left? The Samskaras, the impressions. When a large number of these impressions is left on the mind, they coalesce and become a habit. It is said, "Habit is second nature of man; everything that we are is the result of habit. That gives us consolation, because, if it is only habit, we can make and unmake it at any time.

The Samskaras are left by these vibrations passing out of our mind, each one of them leaving its result. Our character is the sum total of these marks, and according as some particular wave prevails one takes that tone. If good prevails, one becomes good; if wickedness, one becomes wicked; if joyfulness, one becomes happy.

The only remedy for bad habits is counter habits; all the bad habits that have left their impressions are to be controlled by good habits. Go on doing good, thinking holy thoughts continuously; that is the only way to suppress base impressions. Never say any man is hopeless, because he only represents a character, a bundle of habits, which can be checked by new and better ones. Character is repeated habits, and repeated habits alone can reform character.

तत्र स्थितौ यत्नोऽभ्यासः ॥13॥

Continuous struggle to keep them (the Vrittis) perfectly restrained is practice.

What is practice? The attempt to restrain the mind in Chitta form, to prevent its going out into waves.

सतु दीर्घकालनैरन्त्तर्यसत्कारासेवितो दृढभूमिः ॥14॥

It becomes firmly grounded by long constant efforts with great love (for the end to be attained).

Restraint does not come one day, but by long continued practice.

दृष्टानुश्रविकविषयवितृष्णस्य वशीकारसंज्ञावैराग्यम् ॥15॥

That effect which comes to those who have given up their thirst after objects, either seen or heard, and which wills to control the objects, is non-attachment.

The two motive powers of our actions are : (1) what we see ourselves, (2) the experience of others. These two forces throw the mind, the lake, into various waves. Renunciation is the power of battling against these forces and holding the mind in check. Their renunciation is what we want.

I am passing through a street, and a man comes and takes away my watch. That is my own experience. I see it myself, and it immediately throws my Chitta into a wave, taking the form of anger. Allow not that to come. If you cannot prevent that, you are nothing; if you can, you have Vairagya.

Again, the experience of the worldly-minded teaches us that sense-enjoyments are the highest ideal. These are tremendous temptations. To deny them, and not allow the mind to come to a wave form with regard to them is renunciation; to control the twofold motive powers arising from my own experience and from the experience of others, and thus prevent the Chitta from being governed by them is Vairagya. These should be controlled by me, and not by them. This sort of mental strength is called renunciation. Vairagya is the only way to freedom.

तत्परं पुरुषख्यातेर्गुणवैतृष्ण्यम् ॥16॥

That is extreme non-attachment which gives up even the qualities, and comes from the knowledge of (the real nature of) the Purusha.

It is the highest manifestation of the power of Vairagya when it takes away even our attraction towards the qualities. We have first to understand what the Pursuha, the Self is, and what the qualities are.

According to yoga philosophy, the whole of nature consists of three qualities or forces; one is called Tamas, another Rajas, and the third Sattva. These three qualities manifest themselves in the physical world as darkness or inactivity, attraction or repulsion and equilibrium of the two. Everything is in nature. All manifestations are combinations and recombinations of these three forces.

Nature has been divided into various categories by the Sankhyas; the Self of man is beyond all these, beyond nature. It is effulgent, pure and perfect. Whatever of intelligence we see in nature is but the reflection of this Self upon nature. Nature itself is insentient. You must remember that the word Nature also includes the mind; mind is in nature; thought is in nature; from thought, down to the grossest form of matter, everything is in nature, the manifestation of nature. This nature has covered the Self of man, and when nature takes away the covering, the Self appears in its own glory.

The non-attachment, as described in aphorism 15 (as being control of objects or nature) is the greatest help towards manifesting the Self. The next aphorism defines Samadhi, perfect concentration, which is the goal of the yogi.

वितर्कविचारानन्दास्मितानुगमात् सम्प्रज्ञातः ॥17॥

The concentration called right knowledge is that which is followed by reasoning, discrimination, bliss, unqualified egoism.

Samadhi is divided into two varieties. One is called the Samprajnata, and the other the Asamprajnta. In the Samprajnata Samadhi come all the powers of controlling nature. It is of four varieties. The first variety is called the Savitarka, when the mind meditates upon an object again and again by isolating it from other objects.

There are two sorts of objects for meditation in the

twenty-five categories of the Sankhyas; 1) the twenty-five insentient categories of nature, and 2) the one sentient Purusha. This part of yoga is based entirely on Sankhya philosophy. Egoism and will and mind have a common basis, the Chitta or the mind-stuff, out of which they are all manufactured. The mind-stuff takes in the forces of nature, and projects them as thought.

There must be something, again, where both force and matter are one. This is called Avyakta, the unmanifested state of nature before creation, and to which, after the end of a cycle, the whole of nature returns, to come out again after another period. Beyond that is the Purusha, essence of intelligence. Knowledge is power, and as soon as we begin to know a thing, we get power over it; so also when the mind begins to meditate on the different elements, it gains power over them.

That sort of meditation where the external gross elements are the objects is called Savitark.Vitarka means question; Savitarka, with question, questioning the elements, as it were, that may give their truths and their powers to the man who meditates upon them.

There is no liberation in getting powers. It is a wordly search after enjoyments, and there is no enjoyment in this life; all search for enjoyments is vain; that is the old, old lesson which man finds so hard to learn. When he does learn it, he gets out of the universe and becomes free. The possession of what are called occult powers is only intensifying the world, and in the end, intensifying suffering. Though as a scientist, Patanjali is bound to point out the possibilities of this science, he never misses an opportunity to warn us against these powers.

Again, in the very same meditation, when one struggles to take the elements out of time and space, and think of them as they are, it is called Nirvitarka, without question. When the meditation goes a step higher, and takes as in time and space, it is called Savichara, with discrimination; and when in the same meditation one eliminates time and space, and thinks of the fine elements as they are, it is called Nirvichara, without discrimination.

The next step is when the elements are given up, both gross and fine, and the object of meditation is the interior organ, the thinking organ. When the thinking organ is thought of as bereft of the qualities of activity and dullness, it is then called Sananda, the blissful Samadhi.

When the mind itself is the object of meditation, when meditation becomes very ripe and concentrated, when all ideals of the gross and fine materials are given up. When the Sattva state only of the ego remains, but differentiated from all other objects, it is called Sasmita Samadhi. The man who has attained to this has attained to what is called in the Vedas "bereft of body." He can think of himself as without his gross body; but he will have to think of himself as with a fine body. Those that in this state get merged in nature without attaining the goal are called Prakritilayas, but those who do not stop even there reach the goal, which is freedom.

विरामप्रत्ययाभ्यासपूर्वः संस्कारशेषोऽन्यः ॥18॥

There is another Samadhi which is attained by the constant practice of cessation of all mental activity, in which the Chitta retains only the unmanifested impressions.

This is the perfect super-conscious Asamprajnata Samadhi, the state which gives us freedom. The first state does not give us freedom, does not liberate the soul. A man may attain to all powers, and yet fall again. There is no safeguard until the soul goes beyond nature. It is very difficult to do so, although the method seems easy. The method is to meditate on the mind itself, and whenever thought comes, to strike it down, allowing no thought to come into the mind, thus making it an entire vacuum. When we can really do this, that very moment we shall attain liberation.

When persons without training and preparation try to make their minds vacant, they are likely to succeed only in covering themselves with Tamas, the material of ignorance, which makes the mind dull and stupid, and leads them to think that they are making a vacuum of the mind. To be able to really do that is to manifest the greatest strength, the highest control.

When this state Asamprajnata, super-consciousness, is reached, the Samadhi becomes seedless. What is meant by that? In a concentration where there is consciousness, where the mind succeeds only in quelling the waves in the Chitta and holding them down, the waves remain in the form of tendencies. These tendencies (of seeds) become waves again, when the time comes. But when you have destroyed all these tendencies, almost destroyed the mind, then the Samadhi becomes seedless, there are no more seeds in the mind out of which to manufacture again and again this plant of life, this ceaseless round of birth and death.

You may ask, what state would that be in which there is no mind, there is no knowledge?

What we call knowledge is a lower state than the one beyond knowledge. You must always bear in mind that the extremes look very much alike. If a very low vibration of ether is taken as darkness, an intermediate state as light, very high vibration will be darkness again. Similarly, ignorance is the lowest state, knowledge is the highest state, the two extremes of which seem the same. Knowledge itself is a manufactured something, a combination; it is not reality. What is the result of constant practice of this higher concentration?

All old tendencies of restlessness and dullness will be destroyed, as well as the tendencies of goodness too. The case is similar to that of the chemicals used to take the dirt and alloy off gold. When the ore is smelted down, the dross is burnt along with the chemicals. So this constant controlling power will stop the previous bad tendencies, and eventually, the good ones also. Those good and evil tendencies will suppress each other, leaving alone the soul in its own splendour, untrammelled by either good or bad, the omnipresent. omnipotent, and omniscient.

Then the man will know that he had neither birth nor death, nor need of heaven or earth. He will know that he neither came nor went, it was nature which was moving and that movement was reflected upon the soul. The form of the light reflected by the glass upon the wall moves, and the wall foolishly thinks it is moving. So with all of us; it is the Chitta constantly moving making itself into various forms, and we think that we are these various forms. All these delusions will vanish.

When that free soul will command—not pray or beg, but command—then whatever It wants It will be immediately fulfilled; whatever It wants It will be able to do.

According to the Sankhya philosophy, there is no God. It says that there can be no God of this universe, because if there were one, He must be a soul, and a soul must be either bound or free. How can thc soul that is bound by nature, or controlled by nature, create?

It is itself a slave. On the other hand, why should the soul that is free, create and manipulate all these things? It has no desires, so it cannot have any need to create. Secondly, it says the theory of God is an unnecessary one; nature explains all. What is the use of any God? But Kapila teaches that there are many souls, who, though nearly attaining perfection, fall short because they cannot perfectly renounce all powers. Their minds for a time merge in nature, to re-emerge as its masters. Such gods there are.

We shall all become such gods, and according to the Sankhyas, the God spoken of in the Vedas really means one of these free souls. Beyond them there is not an eternally free and blessed Creator of the universe. On the other hand, the yogis say, "Not so, there is a God, there is one Soul separate from all other creation, the ever free, the Teacher of all teachers."

The yogis admit that those, whom the Sankhyas call "the merged in nature," also exist. They are yogis who have fallen short of perfection, and though, for a time debarred from attaining the goal, remain as rulers of parts of the universe.

भव-प्रत्ययो विदेह-प्रकृतिलयानाम् ॥19॥

(This samadhi when not followed by extreme non-attachment) becomes the cause of the re-manifestation of the gods and of those that become merged in nature.

The gods in the Indian systems of philosophy represent certain high offices which are filled successively by various souls. But none of them is perfect.

श्रद्धा-वीर्य-स्मृति-समाधि-प्रज्ञा-पूर्वक इतरेषाम् ॥20॥

To others (this Samadhi) comes through faith, energy, memory, concentration, and discrimination of the real.

These are they who do not want the position of gods or even that of rulers of cycles. They attain to liberation.

तीव्रसंवेगानामासन्नः ॥21॥

Success is speedy for the extremely energetic.

मृदुमध्याधिमात्रत्वात्ततोऽपि विशेषः ॥22॥

The success of yogis differs according as the means they adopt are mild, medium, or intense.

ईश्वरप्रणिधानाद्वा ॥23॥

Or by devotion to Ishvara.

क्लेशकर्मविपाकाशयैरपरामृष्टः पुरुषविशेष ईश्वरः ॥24॥

Ishvara (the supreme Ruler) is a special Purusha, untouched by misery, actions, their results, and desires.

We must again remember that the Patanjala yoga philosophy is based upon the Sankhya philosophy; only in the latter there is no place for God, while with the yogis God has a place. The yogis, however, do not mention many ideas about God, such as creating. God as the creator of the universe is not meant by the Ishvara of yogis. According to the Vedas, Ishvara is the Creator of the universe; because it is harmonious, it must be the manifestation of one will. The yogis want to establish a God, but they arrive at Him in a peculiar fashion of their own. They say:

तत्र निरतिशयं सर्वज्ञत्वबीजम् ॥25॥

In Him becomes infinite that all-knowingness which in others is (only) a germ.

The mind must always travel between two extremes. You can think of limited space, but that very idea gives you also unlimited space. Close your eyes and think of a little space; at the same time that you perceive the little circle, you have a circle round it of unlimited dimensions. It is the same with time. Try to think of a second; you will have, with the same act of perception, to think of time which is unlimited. So with knowledge. Knowledge is only a germ in man but you will have to think of infinite knowledge around it, so that the very constitution of our mind shows us that there is unlimited knowledge, and the yogis call that unlimited knowledge God.

स पूर्वेषामपि गुरुः कालेनानवच्छेदात् ॥26॥

He is the Teacher of even the ancient teachers, being not limited by time.

It is true that all knowledge is within ourselves, but this has to be called forth by another knowledge. Although the capacity to know is inside us, it must be called out, and that calling out of knowledge can only be done, a yogi maintains, through another knowledge. Dead, insentient matter never calls out knowledge, it is the action of knowledge that brings out knowledge. Knowing beings must be with us to call forth what is in us, so these teachers were always necessary.

The world was never without them, and no knowledge can come without them. God is the Teacher of all teachers, because these teachers, however great they may have been—gods or angels—were all bound and limited by time, while God is not. There are two peculiar deductions of the yogis. The first is that in thinking of the limited, the mind must think of the unlimited; and that if one part of that perception is true, so also must the other be, for the reason that their value as perceptions of the mind is equal.

The very fact that man has a little knowledge, shows that God has unlimited knowledge. If I am to take one, why not the other? Reason forces me to take both or reject both. If I believe that there is a man with a litttle knowledge, I must also admit that there is someone behind him with unlimited knowledge. The second deduction is that no knowledge can come without a teacher. It is true as the modern philosophers say, that there is something in man which evolves out of him; all knowledge is in man, but certain environments are necessary to call it out.

We cannot find any knowledge without teachers. If there are men teachers, god teachers or angel teachers, they are all limited; who was the teacher before them? We are forced to admit, as a last conclusion, one teacher, who is not limited by time; and that one Teacher of infinite knowledge, without beginning or end, is called God.

तस्य वाचकः प्रणवः ॥27॥

His manifesting word is Om.

Every idea that you have in the mind has a counterpart in a word; the word and the thought are inseparable. The external part of one and the same thing is what we call word, and the internal part is what we call thought. No man can, by analysis, separate thought from word. The idea that language was created by men—certain men sitting together and deciding upon words, has been proved to be wrong. So long as man has existed there have been words and language.

What is the connection between an idea and a word? Although we see that there must always be a word with a thought, it is not necessary that the same thought requires the same word. The thought may be the same in twenty different countries, yet the language is different. We must have a word to express each thought, but these words need not necessarily have the same sound. Sounds will vary in different nations. Our commentator says. "Although the relation between thought and word is perfectly natural, yet it does not mean a rigid connection between one sound and one idea." These sounds vary, yet the relation between the sounds and the thoughts is a natural one.

The connection between thoughts and sounds is good only if there be a real connection between the thing signified and the symbol; until then that symbol will never come into general use. A symbol is the manifester of the thing signified, and if the thing signified has already an existence, and if, by experience, we know that the symbol has expressed that thing many times, then we are sure that there is a real relation between them. Even if the things are not present, there will be thousands who will know them by their symbols.

There must be a natural connection between the symbol and the thing signified; then, when that symbol is pronounced, it recalls the thing signified. The commentator says the manifesting word of God is Om. Why does he emphasise this word? There are hundreds of words for God. One thought is connected with a thousand words; the idea "God" is connected with hundreds of words, and each one stands as a symbol for God.

This is very good, but there must be a generalisa-tion among all these words, some substratum, some common ground of all these symbols, and that which is the common symbol will be the best, and will really represent them all. In making a sound we use the larynx and the palate as a sounding board. Is there any material sound of which all other sounds must be manifestations, one which is the most natural sound?

Om (Aum) is such a sound, the basis of all sound. The first letter, *A* is the root sound, the key, pronounced without touching any part of the tongue of palate; *M* represents the last sound in the series, being produced by the closed lips, and the *U* rolls from the very root to the end of the sounding board of the mouth. Thus, Om represents the whole phenomena of sound-producing. As such, it must be the natural symbol, the matrix of all the various sounds. It denotes the whole range and possibility of all the words that can be made.

Apart from these speculations, we see that around this word Om are centred all the different religious ideas in India; all the various religious ideas of the Vedas have gathered themselves round this word Om. What has that to do with America and England or any other country? Simply this, that the word has been retained at every stage of religious growth in India, and it has been manipulated to mean all the various ideas about God.

Monists, dualists, monodualists, separatists, and even

atheists took up this Om. Om has become the one symbol for the religious aspiration of the vast majority of human beings. Take, for instance, the English word God. It covers only a limited function, and if you go beyond it, your have to add adjectives, to make it personal, or impersonal, or Absolute God. So with the words for God in every other language; their signification is very small. This word Om, however, has around it all the various significance. As such it should be accepted by everyone.

तज्जपस्तदर्थभावनम् ॥28॥

The repetition of this (Om) and meditating on its meaning (is the way).

Why should there be repetition? We have not forgotten the theory of Samskaras, that the sum total of impressions lives in the mind. They become more and more latent but remain there and as soon as they get the right stimulus, they come out. Molecular vibration never ceases. When this universe is destroyed, all the massive vibrations disappear; the sun, the moon, stars and the earth melt down; but the vibrations remain in the atoms. Each atom performs the same function as the big worlds do. So even when the vibrations of the Chitta subside, its molecular vibrations go on, and when they get the impulse, come out again.

We can now understand what is meant by repetition. It is the greatest stimulus that can be given to the spiritual Samskaras. "One moment of company with the holy makes a ship to cross this ocean of life." Such is the power of association. So this repetition of Om, and thinking of its meaning, is keeping good company in your own mind. Study, and then meditate on what you have studied. Thus light will come to you, the Self will become manifest.

But one must think of Om, and of its meaning too. Avoid evil company, because the scars of old wounds are in you, and evil company is just the thing that is necessary to call them out. In the same way, we are told that good company will call out the good impressions that are in us, but which have become latent. There is nothing holier in the world than to keep good company, because the good impressions will then tend to come to the surface.

ततः प्रत्यकचेतनाधिगमोऽप्यन्तरायाभावश्च ॥29॥

From that is gained (the knowledge of) introspection, and the destruction of obstacles.

The first manifestation of the repetition and thinking of Om is that the introspective power will manifest more and more, all the mental and physical obstacles will begin to vanish. What are the obstacles to the yogi?

व्याधि-स्त्यान-संशय-प्रमादालस्याविरति-भ्रान्तिदर्शनालब्धभूमिकत्वानवस्थितत्वानि चित्तविक्षेपास्तेऽन्तरायाः ॥30॥

Disease, mental laziness, doubt, lack of enthusiasm, lethargy, clinging to sense-enjoyment, false perception, non-attaining concentration, and falling away from the state when obtained, are the obstructing distractions.

Disease: This body is the boat which will carry us to the other shore of the ocean of life. It must be taken care of. Unhealthy persons cannot be yogis. Mental laziness makes us lose all lively interest in the subject, without which there will neither be the will not the energy to practice. Doubts will arise in the mind about the truth of the science, however strong one's intellectual conviction may be, until peculiar psychic experiences come, as hearing or seeing at a distance, etc. These glimpses strengthen the mind and make the student persevere.

Falling away from the state when obtained: Some days or weeks when your are practising, the mind will be calm and easily concentrated, and you will find yourself progressing fast. All of a sudden the progress will stop one day, and you will find yourself, as it were, stranded. Persevere. All progress proceeds by such rise and fall.

दुःख-दौर्मनस्याङ्गमेजयत्व-श्वासप्रश्वासाविक्षेपसहभुवः ॥31॥

Grief, mental distress, tremor of the body, irregular breathing accompany non-retention of concentration.

Concentration will bring perfect repose to mind and body every time it is practised. When the practice has been misdirected, or not enough controlled, these disturbances come. Repetition of Om and self-surrender to the Lord will strengthen the mind, and bring fresh energy. The nervous shakings will come to almost everyone. Do not mind them at all, but keep on practising. Practice will cure them, and make the seat firm.

तत्प्रतिषेधार्थमेकतत्त्वाभ्यासः ॥32॥

To remedy this, the practice of one subject (should be made).

Making the mind take the form of one object for some time will destroy these obstacles. This is general advise. In the following aphorisms it will be expanded and particularised. As one practice cannot suit everyone, various methods will be advanced, and everyone by actual experience will find out that which helps him most.

मैत्री-करुणामुदितोपेक्षाणां सुखदुःखपुण्यापुण्य-विषयाणां भावनातश्चित्त-प्रसादनम् ॥33॥

Friendship, mercy, gladness, and indifference, being thought of in regard to subjects, happy, unhappy, good, and evil respectively, pacify the Chitta.

We must have these four sorts of ideas. We must have friendship for all; we must be merciful towards those that are in misery; when people are happy, we ought to be happy; and to the wicked we must be indifferent. So with all subjects that come before us. If the subject is a good one, we shall feel friendly towards it; if the subject of thought is one that is miserable we must be merciful towards it. If it is good, we must be glad; if it is evil, we must be indifferent. These attitudes of the mind towards the different subjects that come before it will make the mind peaceful.

Most of our difficulties in our daily lives come from being unable to hold our minds in this way. For instance, if a man does evil to us, instantly we want to react evil, and every reaction of evil shows that we are not able to hold the Chitta down; it comes out in waves towards the object, and we lose our power. Every reaction in the form of hatred or evil is so much loss to the mind; and every evil thought or deed of hatred, or any thought of reaction, if it is controlled, will be laid in our favour. It is not that we lose by thus restraining ourselves; we are gaining infinitely more than we suspect. Each time we suppress hatred, or a feeling of anger, it is so much good energy stored up in our favour; that piece of energy will be converted into the higher powers.

प्रच्छर्दन-विधारणाभ्यां वा प्राणस्य ॥34॥

By throwing out and restraining the Breath.

The word used is Prana. **The Prana is not exactly breath. It is the name for the energy that is in the universe.** Whatever you see in the universe, whatever moves or works, or has life, is a manifestation of the Prana. The sum total of the energy displayed in the universe is called Prana. This Prana, before a cycle begins, remains in an almost motionless state; and when the cycle begins, this Prana begins to manifest itself. It is this Prana that is manifested as motion—as the nervous motion in human beings or animals; and the same Prana is manifesting as thought and so on.

The whole universe is a combination of Prana and Akasha; so is the human body. Out of Akasha you get the different materials that you feel and see, and out of Prana all the various forces. Now this throwing out and restraining the Prana is what is called Pranayama. Patanjali, the father of the yoga philosophy, does not give very many particular directions about Pranayama, but later on, other yogis found out various things about this Pranayama and made of it a great science.

With Patanjali it is one of the many ways, but he does not lay much stress on it. He means that you simply throw the air out, and draw it in, and hold it for some time, that is all, and by that, the mind will become a little calmer. But, later on, you will find that out of this is evolved a particular science called Pranayama. We shall hear a little of what these later yogis have to say.

Prana is not the breath; but that which causes the motion of the breath, that which is the vitality of the breath is the Prana.

Again the word Prana is used for all the senses; they are all called Pranas, the mind is called Prana; and so we see that Prana is force. And yet we cannot call it force, because force is only the manifestation of it. It is that which manifests itself as force and everything else in the way of motion. The Chitta, the mind-stuff, is the engine which draws in the Prana from the surroundings, and manufactures out of Prana the various vital forces—those that keep the body in preservation—and thought, will, and all other powers.

By the above mentioned process of breathing we can control all the various motions in the body, and the various nerve currents that are running through the body. First we begin to recognize them, and then we slowly get control over them.

These later yogis consider that there are three main

currents of this Prana in the human body. One they call Ida, another Pingala, and the third Sushumna. Pingala, according to them, is on the right side of the spinal column, and the Ida on the left, and in the middle of the spinal column is the Sushumna, an empty channel. Ida and Pingala, according to them, are the currents working in every man, and through these currents, we are performing all the functions of life. Sushumna is present in all, as a possibility; but it works only in the yogi.

You must remember that yoga changes the body. As you go on practising, your body changes; it is not the same body that you had before the practice. That is very rational, and can be explained, because every new thought that we have must make, as it were, a new channel through the brain, and that explains the tremendous conservatism of human nature.

Human nature likes to run through the ruts that are already there, because it is easy. If we think, just for example's sake, that the mind is like a needle, and the brain substance a soft lump before it, then each thought that we have makes a street, as it were, in the brain, and this street would close up, but for the grey matter which comes and makes a lining to keep it separate.

If there were no grey matter, there would be no memory, because memory means going over these old streets, retracing a thought as it were; Now perhaps you have marked that when one talks on subjects in which one takes a few ideas that are familiar to everyone, and combines and recombines them, it is easy to follow because these channels are present in everyone's brain, and it is only necessary to recur to them. But whenever a new subject comes, new channels have to be made, so it is not understood readily. And that is why the brain (it is the brain, and not the people themselves) refuses unconsciously to be acted upon by new ideas. It resists.

The Prana is trying to make new channels, and the brain will not allow it. This is the secret of conservatism. The fewer channels there have been in the brain, and the less the needle of the Prana has made these passages, the more conservative will be the brain, the more it will struggle against new thoughts. The more thoughtful the man, the more complicated will be the streets in his brain, and the more easily he will take to new ideas, and understand them.

So with every fresh idea, we make a new impression in the brain, cut new channels through the brain-stuff, and that is why we find that in the practice of yoga (it being an entirely new set of thoughts and motives) there is so much physical resistance at first. That is why we find that the part of religion which deals with the world-side of nature is so widely accepted, while the other part, the Philosophy, or the Psychology, which deals with the inner nature of man, is so frequently neglected.

We must remember the definition of this world of ours; it is only the Infinite Existence projected into the plane of consciousness. A little of the Infinite is projected into consciousness, and that we call our world. So there is an Infinite beyond; and religion has to deal with both—with the little lamp we call our world, and with the Infinite beyond.

Any religion which deals with one only of these two will be defective. It must deal with both. The part of religion which deals with the part of the Infinite which has come into the plane of consciousness, got itself caught, as it were, in the plane of consciousness, in the cage of time, space, and causation, is quite familiar to us, because we are in that already, and ideas about this world have been with us almost from time immemorial.

The part of religion which deals with the Infinite beyond comes entirely new to us, and getting ideas about it produces new channels in the brain, disturbing the whole system, and that is why you find in the practice of yoga ordinary people are at first turned out of their grooves. In order to lessen these disturbances as much as possible, all these methods are devised by Patanjali, that we may practise any one of them best suited to us.

विषयवती वा प्रवृत्तिरुत्पन्ना मनसः स्थितिनिबन्धिनी ॥35॥

Those forms of concentration that bring extraordinary sense-perceptions cause perseverance of mind.

This naturally comes with Dharana, concentration; the yogis say, if the mind becomes concentrated on the tip of the nose, one begins to smell, after a few days, wonderful perfumes. If it becomes concentrated at the root of the tongue, one begins to hear sounds; if on the tip of the tongue, one begins to taste wonderful flavours; if on the middle of the tongue, one feels as if one were coming in contact with something.

If one concentrates one's mind on the palate, one begins to see peculiar things. If a man whose mind is disturbed wants to take up some of these practices of yoga, yet doubts the truth of them, he will have his doubts set at rest when, after a little practice, these things come to him, and he will persevere.

विशोका वा ज्योतिष्मती ॥36॥

Or (by the meditation on) the Effulgent Light, which is beyond all sorrow.

This is another sort of concentration. Think of the lotus of the heart, with petals downwards, and running through it, the Sushumna; take in the breath, and while throwing the breath out imagine that the lotus is turned with the petals upwards, and inside that lotus is an effulgent light. Meditate on that.

वीतरागविषयं वा चित्तम् ॥37॥

Or (by meditation on) the heart that has given up all attachment to sense-objects.

Take some holy person, some great person whom you revere, some saint whom you know to be perfectly non-attached, and think of his heart. That heart has become non-attached, and meditate on the heart; it will calm the mind. If you cannot do that, there is the next way.

स्वप्ननिद्राज्ञानालम्बनं वा ॥38॥

Or by meditating on the knowledge that comes in sleep.

Sometimes a man dreams that he has seen angels coming to him and talking to him, that he is in an ecstatic condition. That he has heard music floating through the air. He is in a blissful condition in that dream, and when he wakes, it makes a deep impression on him. Think of that dream as real, and meditate upon it. If you cannot do that, meditate on any holy thing that pleases you.

यथाभिमतध्यानाद्वा ॥39॥

Or by the meditation on anything that appeals to one as good.

This does not mean any wicked subjects, but anything good that you like, any place that you like best, any scenery that you like best, any idea that you like best, anything that will concentrate the mind.

परमाणु-परममहत्त्वान्तोऽस्य वशीकारः ॥40॥

The yogi's mind thus meditating becomes unobstructed from the atomic to the infinite.

The mind, by this practice, easily contemplates the most minute as well as the biggest thing. Thus the mind-waves become fainter.

क्षीणवृत्तेरभिजातस्येव मणेर्ग्रहीतृ-ग्रहण-ग्राह्येषु तत्स्थतदञ्जनता समापत्तिः ॥41॥

The yogi whose Vrittis have thus become powerless (controlled) obtains in the receiver (the instrument of) receiving, and the received (the Self, the mind, and external objects), concentratedness and sameness, like the crystal (before different coloured objects).

What results from this constant meditation? We must remember how in a previous aphorism Patanjali went into the various states of meditation, how the first would be the gross, the second the fine, and from them the advance was to still finer objects. The result of these meditations is that we can meditate as easily on the fine as on the gross objects, Here the yogi sees the three things, the receiver, the received, and the receiving instrument, corresponding to the soul, external objects, and the mind.

There are three objects of meditation given us. First, the gross things, as bodies, or material objects; second, fine things, as the mind, the Chitta; and third, the Purusha qualified, not the Purusha itself, but the Egoism. By practice, the yogi gets established in all these meditations. Whenever he meditates he can keep out all other thoughts he becomes identified with that on which he meditates. When he meditates, he is like a piece of crystal. Before flowers the crystal becomes almost identified with the flowers. If the flower is red, the crystal looks red, or if the flower is blue, the crystal looks blue.

तत्र शब्दार्थज्ञानविकल्पैः सङ्कीर्णा सवितर्का समापत्तिः ॥42॥

Sound, meaning, and resulting knowledge, being mixed up, is (called) Samadhi with question.

Sound here means vibration, meaning the nerve currents which conduct it; and knowledge, reaction. All the various meditations we have had so far, Patanjali calls Savitarka (meditation with question). Later on he gives us higher and higher Dhyanas. In these that are called "with question," we keep the quality of subject and object, which results from the mixture of word, meaning, and knowledge.

There is first the external vibration, the word. This carried inward by the sense currents, is the meaning. After that there comes a reactionary wave in the Chitta, which is knowledge, but the mixture of these three makes up what we call knowledge. In all the meditations up to this we get this mixture as objects of meditation. The next Samadhi is higher.

स्मृतिपरिशुद्धौ स्वरूपशून्येवार्थमात्रनिर्भासा निर्वितर्का ॥43॥

The Samadhi called "without question" (comes) when the memory is purified, or devoid of qualities, expressing only the meaning (of the meditated object).

It is by the practice of meditation of these three that we come to the state where these three do not mix. We can get rid of them. We will first try to understand what these three are. Here is the Chitta; you will always remember the smile of the mind-stuff to a lake and the vibration, the word, the sound, like a pulsation coming over it. You have that calm lake in you, and I pronounce a word, "Cow". As soon as it enters through your ears there is a wave produced in your Chitta along with it. So that wave represents the idea of the cow, the form or the meaning as we call it. The apparent cow that you know is really the waves in the mind-stuff that comes as a reaction to the internal and external sound vibration. With the sound, the wave dies away; it can never exist without a word.

You may ask how it is, when we only think of the cow, and do not hear a sound. You make that sound yourself. You are saying "cow" faintly in your mind, and with that comes a wave. There cannot be any wave without this impulse of sound; and when it is not from outside, it is from inside and when the sound dies, the wave dies. What remains? The result of the reaction, and that is knowledge. These three are so closely combined in our mind that we cannot separate them. When the sound comes, the senses vibrate, and the wave rises in reaction; they follow so closely upon one another that there is no discerning one from the other.

When this meditation has been practised for a long time, memory, the receptacle of all impressions, becomes purified, and we are able clearly to distinguish them from one another. This is called Nirvitarka, concentration without question.

एतयैव सविचारा निर्विचारा च सूक्ष्मविषया व्याख्याता ॥44॥

By this process, (the concentrations) with discrimination and without discrimination, whose objects are finer, are (also) explained.

A process similar to the preceding is applied again; only the objects to be taken up in the former meditation are gross; in this they are fine.

सूक्ष्मविषयत्वञ्चालिङ्ग-पर्यवसानम् ॥45॥

The finer objects end with the Pradhana.

The gross objects are only the elements and everything manufactured out of them. The fine objects begin with the Tanmatras or fine particles. The organs, the mind, egoism, the mind-stuff (the cause of all manifestaion), the equilibrium state of Sattva, Rajas, and Tamas materials—called Pradhana (chief), Prakriti (nature), or Avyakta (unmanifest)— are all included within the category of fine objects, the Purusha (the soul) alone being excepted.

ता एव सबीजः समाधिः ॥46॥

These concentrations are with seed.

These do not destroy the seeds of past actions, and thus cannot give liberation, but what they bring to the yogi is stated in the following aphorism.

निर्विचार-वैशारद्येऽध्यात्मप्रसादः ॥47॥

The concentration "without discrimination" being purified, the Chitta becomes firmly fixed.

ऋतम्भरा तत्र प्रज्ञा ॥48॥

The knowledge in that is called "filled with Truth."

The next aphorism will explain this.

श्रुतानुमानप्रज्ञाभ्यामन्यविषया विशेषार्थत्वात् ॥49॥

The knowledge that is gained from testimony and inference is about common objects. That from the Samadhi just mentioned is of a much higher order, being able to penetrate where inference and testimony cannot go.

The idea is that we have to get our knowledge of ordinary objects by direct perception and by inference therefrom, and from testimony of people who are competent. By "people who are competent", the yogis always mean the Rishis, or the Seers of the thoughts recorded in the scriptures—the Vedas. According to them, the only proof of the scriptures is that they were the testimony of competent persons, yet they say the scriptures cannot take us to realisation. We can read all the Vedas, and yet will not realise anything, but when we practise their teachings, then we attain to that state which realises what the scriptures say, which penetrates where neither reason nor perception nor inference can go, and where the testimony of others cannot avail. This is what is meant by the aphorism.

Realisation is real religion, all the rest is only preparation—hearing lectures, or reading books, or reasoning is merely preparing the ground; it is not religion. Intellectual assent and intellectual dissent are not religion. The central idea of the yogis is that just as we come in direct contact with objects of the senses, so religion even can be directly perceived in a far more intense sense.

The truths of religion, as God and Soul, cannot be perceived by the external senses. I cannot see God with my eyes, not can I touch Him with my hands, and we also know that neither can we reason beyond the senses. Reason leaves us at a point quite indecisive; we may reason all our lives, as the world has been doing for thousands of years, and the result is that we find we are incompetent to prove or disprove the facts of religion. What we perceive directly we take as the basis, and upon that basis we reason. So it is obvious that reasoning has to run within these bounds of perception. It can never go beyond.

The whole scope of realisation, therefore, is beyond sense-perception. The yogis say that man can go beyond his direct sense-perception, and beyond his reason also. Man has in him the faculty, the power of transcending even his intellect, a power which is in every being, every creature. By the practice of yoga that power is aroused , and then man transcends the ordinary limits of reason, and directly perceives things which are beyond all reason.

तज्जः संस्कारोऽन्यसंस्कारप्रतिबन्धी ॥50॥

The resulting impression from this Samadhi obstructs all other impressions.

We have seen in the foregoing aphorism that the only way of attaining of that super-consciousness is by concentration, and we have also seen, that what hinder the mind from concentration are the past Samskaras, impressions. All of you have observed that, when you are trying to concentrate your mind, your thoughts wander. When you are trying to think of God, that is the very time these Samskaras appear. At other times they are not so active, but when you want them not, they are sure to be there, trying their best to crowd in your mind.

Why should that be so? Why should they be much more potent at the time of concentration? It is because you are repressing them, and they react with all their force. At other times they do not react. How countless these old past impressions must be, all lodged somewhere in the Chitta, ready, waiting like tigers, to jump up! These have to be suppressed that the one idea which we want may arise, to the exclusion of the others. Instead they are all struggling to come up at the same time.

These are the various powers of the Samskaras in hindering concentration of the mind. So this Samadhi which has just been given is the best to be practised, on account of its power of suppressing the Samskaras. The Samskara which will be raised by this sort of concentration will be so powerful that it will hinder the action of the others and hold them in check.

तस्यापि निरोधे सर्वनिरोधान्निर्बीजः समाधिः ॥51॥

By the restraint of even this (impression, which obstructs all other impressions) all being restrained, comes the "seedless" Samadhi.

You remember that our goal is to perceive the soul itself. We cannot perceive the soul, because it has got mingled up with nature, with the mind, with the body. The ignorant man thinks his body is the Soul. The learned man thinks his mind is the Soul. But both of them are mistaken. What makes the Soul get mingled up with all this? Different waves in the Chitta rise and cover the Soul; we only see a little reflection of the Soul through these waves: so, if the wave is one of anger, we see the Soul as angry. "I am angry," one says. If it is one of love, we see ourselves reflected in that wave, and say we are loving. If that wave is one of weakness, and the Soul is reflected in it, we think we are weak. These various ideas come from these impressions, these Samskaras covering the Soul.

The real nature of the Soul is not perceived as long as there is one single wave in the lake of the Chitta; this real nature will never be perceived until all the waves have subsided. So, first, Patanjali teaches us the meaning of these waves; secondly, the best way to repress them; and thirdly, how to make one wave so strong as to suppress all other waves, fires-eating fire as it were. When only one remains, it will be easy to suppress that also, and when that is gone, this Samadhi or concentration is called seedless. It leaves nothing, and the Soul is manifested just as it is, in its own glory. Then alone we know that the Soul is not a compound; it is the only eternal simple in the universe, and as such, it cannot be born, it cannot die; it is immortal, indestructible, the ever-living essence of intelligence.

2

The Practice of Concentration

तपः-स्वाध्यायेश्वरप्रणिधानानि क्रियायोगः ॥1॥

Mortification, study, and surrendering fruits of work to God are called Kriya-yoga.

The Samadhis with which we ended our last chapter are very difficult to attain; so we must take them up slowly. The first step, the preliminary step, is called Kriyayoga. Literally this means work, working towards yoga. The organs are the horses, the mind is the rein, the intellect is the charioteer, the soul is the rider, and the body is the chariot. The master of the household, the king, the self of man, is sitting in this chariot. If the horses are very strong and do not obey the rein, if the charioteer, the intellect, does not know how to control the horses, then the chariot will come to grief. But if the organs, the horses, are well controlled, and if the rein, the mind, is well held in the hands of the charioteer, the intellect, the chariot reaches the goal.

What is meant, therefore, by this mortification? Holding the rein firmly while guiding the body and the organs; not letting them do anything they like, but keeping them both under proper control. Study. What is meant by study in this case? No study of novels or story books, but study of those works which teach the liberation of the soul. Then again this study does not mean controversial studies at all. The yogi is supposed to have finished his period of controversy. He has had enough of that, and has become satisfied. He only studies to intensify his convictions.

Vada and Siddhanta—these are the two sorts of scriptural knowledge—Vada (the argumentative) and Siddhanta (the decisive). When a man is entirely ignorant he takes up the first of these, the argumentative fighting, and reasoning pro and con; and when he has finished that he takes up the Siddhanta, the decisive, arriving at a conclusion. Simply arriving at this conclusion will not do. It must be intensified.

Books are infinite in number, and time is short; therefore the secret of knowledge is to take what is essential. Take that and try to live up to it. There is an old Indian legend that if you place a cup of milk and water before a Raja-Hamsa (swan), he will take all the milk and leave the water. In that way we should take what is of value in knowledge, and leave the dross. Intellectual gymnastics are necessary at first. We must not go blindly into anything. The yogi has passed the argumentative stage, and has come to a conclusion, which is, like the rock, immovable. The only thing he now seeks to do is to intensify that conclusion. Do not argue, he says; if one forces arguments upon you, be silent. Do not answer any argument, but go away calmly, because arguments only disturb the mind.

The only thing necessary is to train the intellect, what is the use of disturbing it for nothing? The intellect is but a weak instrument, and can give us only knowledge limited by the senses. The yogi wants to go beyond the senses; therefore, intellect is of no use to him. He is certain of this and, therefore, is silent, and does not argue . Every argument throws his mind out of balance, creates a disturbance in the Chitta, and a disturbance is a drawback. Argumentations and searching of the reason are only by the way. There are much higher things beyond them. The whole of life is not for schoolboy fights and debating societies. "Surrendering the fruits of work to God" is to take to ourselves neither credit nor blame, but to give both up to the Lord and be at peace.

समाधि-भावनार्थः क्लेश-तनूकरणार्थश्च ॥2॥

(It is for) the practice of Samadhi and minimising the pain-bearing obstructions.

Most of us make our minds like spoilt children, allowing them to do whatever they want. Therefore it is necessary that Kriyayoga should be constantly practised, in order to gain control of the mind, and bring it into subjection. The obstructions to yoga arise from lack of control, and cause us pain. They can only be removed by denying the mind, and holding it in check, through the means of Kriyayoga.

अविद्यास्मिता-राग-द्वेषाभिनिवेशाः क्लेशाः ॥3॥

The pain-bearing obstructions are— ignorance, egoism, attachment, aversion, and clinging to life.

These are the five pains, the fivefold tie that binds us down, of which ignorance is the cause and the other four its effects. It is the only cause of all our misery. What else can make us miserable? The nature of the soul is eternal bliss. What can make it sorrowful except ignorance, hallucination, delusion? All pain of the Soul is simply delusion.

अविद्याक्षेत्रमुत्तरेषां प्रसुप्त-तनु-विच्छिन्नोदाराणाम् ॥4॥

Ignorance is the productive field of all these that follow, whether they are dormant, attenuated, overpowered, or expanded.

Ignorance is the cause of egoism, attachment, aversion, and clinging to life. These impressions exist in different states. They are sometimes dormant. You often hear the expression "innocent as a baby," yet in the baby may be the state of a demon or of a god, which will come out by degrees. In the yogi, these impressions, the Samskaras left by past actions, are attenuated, that is, exist in a very fine state, and he can control them, and not allow them to become manifest.

"Overpowered" means that sometimes one set of impressions is held down for a while by those that are stronger, but they come out when that repressing cause is removed. The last state is the "expanded," when the Samsaras, having helpful surroundings, attain to a great activity, either as good or evil.

अनित्याशुचि-दुःखानात्मसु नित्यशुचि सुखात्मख्यातिरविद्या ॥5॥

Ignorance is taking the non-eternal, the impure, the painful, and the non-Self for the eternal, the pure, the happy, and the Atman or Self (respectively).

All the different sorts of impressions have one source, ignorance. We have first to learn what ignorance is. All of us think, "I am the body and not the Self, the pure, the effulgent, the ever blissful," and that is ignorance. We think of man, and see man as body. This is the great delusion.

दृगदर्शनशक्त्योरेकात्मतैवास्मिता ॥6॥

Egoism is the identification of the seer with the instrument of seeing.

The seer is really the Self, the pure one, the ever holy, the infinite, the immortal. This is the Self of man. And what are the instruments? The Chitta, or mind-stuff, the Buddhi, determinative faculty, the Manas, or mind, and the Indriyas, or sense-organs. These are the instruments for him to see the external world, and the identification of the Self with the instruments is what is called the ignorance of egoism.

We say, "I am the mind", "I am thought", "I am angry", or "I am happy". How can we be angry and how can we hate? We should identify ourselves with the Self that cannot change. If it is unchangeable, how can it be one moment happy, and one moment unhappy? It is formless, infinite, omnipresent. What can change it? It is beyond all law. What can affect it? Nothing in the universe can produce an effect on it. Yet through ignorance, we identify ourselves with the mind-stuff, and think we feel pleasure or pain.

सुखानुशयी रागः ॥7॥

Attachment is that which dwells on pleasure.

We find pleasure in certain things, and the mind like a current flows towards them; and this following the pleasure centre, as it were, is what is called attachment. We are never attached where we do not find pleasure. We find pleasure in very queer things sometimes, but the principle remains: wherever we find pleasure, there we are attached.

दुःखानुशयी द्वेषः ॥8॥

Aversion is that which dwells on pain.

That which gives us pain we immediately seek to get away from.

स्वरसवाही विदुषोऽपि तथारूढोऽभिनिवेशः ॥9॥

Flowing through its own nature, and established even in the learned, is the clinging to life.

This clinging to life you see manifested in every animal. Upon it many attempts have been made to build the theory of a future life, because men are so fond of life that they desire a future life also. Of course it goes without saying that this argument is without much value, but the most curious part of it is, that, in Western countries, the idea that this clinging to life indicates a possibility of future life applies only to men, but does not include animals. In India this clinging to life has been one of the arguments to prove past experience and existence.

For instance, if it be true that all our knowledge has

come from experience, then it is sure that which we never experienced we cannot imagine or understand. As soon as chickens are hatched they begin to pick up food. Many times it has been seen, where ducks have been hatched by hens, that, as soon as they came out of the eggs they flew to water, and the mother thought they would be drowned. If experience be the only source of knowledge, where did these chickens learn to pick up food, or the ducklings that the water was their natural element? If you say it is instinct, it means nothing—it is simply giving a word, but is no explanation.

What is this instinct? We have many instincts in ourselves. For instance, most of the ladies play the piano, and remember, when she first learnt, how carefully she had to put her fingers on the black and the whites keys, one after the other, but now, after long years of practice, she can talk with her friends while her fingers play mechanically. It has become instinct. So with every work we do; by practice it becomes instinct, it becomes automatic; but so far as we know, all the cases which we now regard as automatic are degenerated reason.

In the language of the yogi, instinct is involved reason. Discrimination becomes involved, and gets to be automatic Samskaras. Therefore, it is perfectly logical to think that all we call instinct in this world is simply involved reason. As reason cannot come without experience, all instinct is, therefore, the result of past experience. Chickens fear the hawk and ducklings love the water; these are both the results of past experience. Then the question is whether that experience belongs to a particular soul, or to the body simply, whether this experience which comes to the duck is the duck's forefather's experience, or the duck's own experience.

Modern scientific men hold that it belongs to the body, but the yogis hold that it is the experience of the mind, transmitted through the body. This is called the theory of reincarnation.

We have seen that all our knowledge whether we call it perception, or reason, or instinct, must come through that one channel called experience, and all that we now call instinct is the result of past experience, degenerated into instinct and that instinct regenerates into reason again. So on throughout the universe, and upon this has been built one of the chief arguments for reincarnation in India. The recurring experiences of various fears, in course of time, produce this clinging to life. That is why the child is instinctively afraid, because the past experience of pain is there in it.

Even in the most learned men, who know that this body will go, and who say "never mind, we have had hundreds of bodies, the soul cannot die"—even in them, with all their intellectual convictions, we still find this clinging on to life. Why is this clinging to life? We have seen that it has become instinctive. In the psychological language of the yogis it has become a Samskara. The Samskaras, fine and hidden, are sleeping in the Chitta. All this past experience of death, all that which we call instinct, is experience become subconscious. It lives in the Chitta, and is not inactive, but is working underneath.

The Chitta-vrittis, the mind-waves, which are gross, we can appreciate and feel; they can be more easily controlled, but what about the finer instincts? How can they be controlled? When I am angry, my whole mind becomes a huge wave of anger. I feel it, see it, handle it, can easily manipulate it, can fight with it; but I shall not succeed perfectly in the fight until I can get down below to its causes.

A man says something very harsh to me, and I begin to feel that I am getting heated, and he goes on till I am perfectly angry and forget myself, identify myself with anger. When he first began to abuse me, I thought, "I am going to be angry". Anger was one thing, and I was another; but when I became angry, I was anger.

These feelings have to be controlled in the germ, the root, in their fine forms, before even we have become conscious that they are acting on us.

With the vast majority of mankind the fine states of these passions are not even known—the states in which they emerge from subconsciousness. When a bubble is rising from the bottom of the lake, we do not see it, nor even when it has nearly come to the surface; it is only when it bursts and makes a ripple that we know it is there. We shall only be successful in grappling with the waves when we can get hold of them in their fine causes, and until you can get hold of them, and subdue them before they become gross, there is no hope of conquering any passion perfectly.

To control our passions we have to control them at their very roots; then alone shall we be able to burn out their very seeds. As fried seeds thrown into the ground will never come up, so these passions will never arise.

ते प्रतिप्रसवहेयाः सूक्ष्माः ॥10॥

The fine Samskaras are to be conquered by resolving them into their causal state.

Samskaras are the subtle impressions that manifest themselves into gross forms later on. How are these fine Samskaras to be controlled?—By resolving the effect into its cause. When the Chitta, which is an effect, is resolved into its cause, Asmita, or Egoism, then only the fine impression die along with it. Meditation cannot destroy these.

ध्यानहेयास्तद्वृत्तयः ॥11॥

By meditation, their (gross) modifications are to be rejected.

Meditation is one of the great means of controlling the

rising of these waves. By meditation you can make the mind subdue these waves, and if you go on practising meditation for days, and months, and years, until it has become a habit, until it will come in spite of yourself, anger and hatred will be controlled and checked.

क्लेशमूलः कर्माशयो दृष्टादृष्टजन्मवेदनीयः ॥12॥

The "receptacle of works" has its root in these pain-bearing obstructions, and their experience is in this visible life, or in the unseen life.

By the "receptacle of works" is meant the sum total of Samskaras. Whatever work we do, the mind is thrown into a wave, and after the work is finished, we think the wave is gone. No, it has only become fine, but it is still there. When we try to remember the work, it comes up again and becomes a wave. So it was there; if not, there would not have been memory. Thus every action, every thought, good or bad, just goes down and becomes fine, and is there stored up.

Both happy and unhappy thoughts are called pain-bearing obstructions, because according to the yogis, they, in the long run, bring pain. All happiness which comes from the senses will eventually, bring pain. All enjoyment will make us thirst for more, and that brings pain as its result. There is no limit to man's desires; he goes on desiring, and when he comes to a point where desire cannot be fulfilled, the result is pain. Therefore, the yogis regard the sum total of the impressions, good or evil, as pain-bearing obstructions; they obstruct the way to freedom of the Soul.

It is the same with the Samskaras, the fine roots of all our works; they are the causes which will again bring effects, either in this life, or in the lives to come. In exceptional cases when these Samskaras are very strong, they bear fruit quickly; exceptional acts of wickedness, or of goodness, bring their fruits even in this life. The yogis hold that men who are able to acquire a tremendous power of good Samskaras do not have to die, but, even in this life, can change their bodies into god-bodies.

There are several such cases mentioned by the yogis in their books. These men change the very material of their bodies; they rearrange the molecules in such fashion that they have no more sickness, and what we call death does not come to them.

Whey should not this be? The physiological meaning of food is assimilation of energy from the sun. The energy has reached the plant, the plant is eaten by an animal, and the animal by men. The science of it is that we take so much energy from the sun, and make it part of ourselves. That being the case, why should there be only one way of assimilating energy?

The plant's way is not the same as ours; the earth's process of assimilating energy differs from our own. But all assimilate energy in some form or other. The yogis say that they are able to assimilate energy by the power of the mind alone, that they can draw in as much of it as they desire without recourse to the ordinary method. As a spider makes its web out of its own substance, and becomes bound in it, and cannot go anywhere except along the lines of that web, so we have projected out of our own substance this network called the nerves, and we cannot work except through the channels of those nerves. The yogi says we need not be bound by that.

Similarly, we can send electricity to only part of the world but we have to send it by means of wires. Nature can send vast masses of electricity without any wires at all. Why cannot we do the same? **We can send mental electricity. What we call mind is very much the same as electricity.** It is clear that this nerve fluid has some amount of electricity, because it is polarised, and it answers all electrical directions. We can only send our electricity through these nerve channels. Why not send the mental electricity without this aid?

The yogis say it is perfectly possible and practicable, and that when you can do that you will work all over the universe. You will be able to work with anybody anywhere, without the help of the nervous system. When the soul is acting through these channels, we say a man is living, and when these cease to work, a man is said to be dead. But when a man is able to act either with or without these channels, birth and death will have no meaning for him. All the bodies in the universe are made up of Tanmatras, their difference lies in the arrangement of the latter. If you are the arranger, you can arrange a body in one way or another.

Who makes up this body but you? Who eats the food? If another ate the food for you, you would not live long. Who makes the blood out of food? You, certainly. Who purifies the blood, and sends it through the veins? You.

We are the masters of the body, and we live in it. Only we have lost the knowledge of how to rejuvenate it. We have become automatic, degenerate. We have forgotten the process of arranging its molecules. So, what we do automatically has to be done knowingly. We are the masters and we have to regulate that arrangement; and as soon as we can do that, we shall be able to rejuvenate just as we like, and then we shall have neither birth nor disease nor death.

सति मूले तद्विपाको जात्यायुर्भोगाः ॥13॥

The root being there, the fruition comes (in the form of) species, life, and experience of pleasure and pain.

The roots, the causes, the Samskaras being there, they manifest and form the effects. The cause dying down becomes the effect: the effect getting subtler becomes the cause of the next effect. A tree bears a seed, which becomes the cause of another tree, and so on. All our works now are the effects of past Samskaras; again, these works becoming Samskaras will be the causes of future actions, and thus we go on. So this aphorism says that the cause being there, the fruit must come, in the form of species of beings; one will be a man, another an angel, another an animal, another a demon.

Then there are different effects of Karma in life. One man lives fifty years, another a hundred, another dies in two years, and never attains maturity; all these difference in life are regulated by past Karma. One man is born, as it were, for pleasure; if he buries himself in a forest, pleasure will follow him there. Another man, wherever he goes, is followed by pain; everything becomes painful for him. It is the result of their own past. According to the philosophy of the yogis, all virtuous actions bring pleasure, and all vicious actions bring pain. Any man who does wicked deeds is sure to reap their fruit in the form of pain.

ते ह्लादपरितापफलाः पुण्यापुण्यहेतुत्वात् ॥14॥

They bear fruit as pleasure or pain, caused by virtue or vice.

परिणामताप-संस्कारदुःखैर्गुणवृत्तिविरोधाच्च दुःखमेव सर्वं विवेकिनः ॥15॥

To the discriminating, all is, as it were, painful on account of everything bringing pain either as consequence, or as anticipation of loss of happiness, or as fresh craving arising from impression of happiness, and also as counteraction of qualities.

The yogis say that the man who has discriminating powers, the man of good sense, sees through all that are called pleasure and pain, and knows that they come to all, and that one follows and melts into the other; he sees that men follow an *ignis fatuus* all their lives, and never succeed in fulfilling their desires.

The great King Yudhishthira once said that the most wonderful thing in life is that every moment we see people dying around us, and yet we think we shall never die. Surrounded by all sorts of experiences of fickleness, we think our love is the only lasting love.

How can that be? Even love is selfish, and the yogi says that in the end we shall find that even the love of husbands and wives, and children and friends, slowly decays. Decadence seizes everything in this life. It is only when everything, even love, fails, that, with a flash, man finds out how vain, how dreamlike is this world. Then he catches a glimpse of Vairagya (renunciation), catches a glimpse of the Beyond. It is only by giving up this world that the other comes; never through holding on to this one.

Never yet was there a great soul who had not to reject sense-pleasures and enjoyments to acquire his greatness. The cause of misery is the clash between the different forces of nature, one dragging one way, and another dragging another, rendering permanent happiness impossible.

हेयं दुःखमनागतम् ॥16॥

The misery which is not yet come is to be avoided.

Some Karma we have worked out already, some we are working out now in the present and some are waiting to bear fruit in the future. The first kind is past and gone. The second we will have to work out, and it is only that which is waiting to bear fruit in the future that we can conquer and control, towards which end all our forces should be directed. This is what Patanjali means when he says that Samskaras are to be controlled by resolving them into their causal state (II.10)

द्रष्टृदृश्ययोः संयोगो हेयहेतुः ॥17॥

The cause of that which is to be avoided is the

junction of the seer and the seen.

Who is the seer? The Self of man, the Purusha. What is the seer? The whole of nature beginning with the mind, down to gross matter. All pleasure and pain arise from the junction between this Purusha and the mind. The Purusha, you must remember, according to this philosophy, is pure; when joined to nature, it appears to feel pleasure or pain by reflection.

प्रकाश-क्रिया-स्थितिशीलं भूतेन्द्रियात्मकं भोगापवर्गार्थं दृश्यम् ॥18॥

The experienced is composed of elements and organs, is of the nature of illumination, action and inertia, and is for the purpose of experience and release (of the experiencer).

The experienced, that is nature, is composed of elements and organs—the elements, gross and fine, which compose the whole of nature, and the organs of the senses, mind, etc.— and is of the nature of illumination (Sattva), action (Rajas), and inertia (Tamas). What is the purpose of the whole of nature? That the Purusha may gain experience. The Purusha has, as it were, forgotten its mighty godly nature.

There is a story that the king of the gods, Indra, once became a pig, wallowing in mire; he had a she-pig, and a lot of baby pigs, and was very happy. Then some gods saw his plight, and came to him, and told him, "You are the king of the gods, you have all the gods under your command. Why are you here?" But Indra said, "Never mind; I am all right here; I do not care for heaven while I have this sow and these little pigs."

The poor gods were at their wits' end. After a time they decided to slay all the pigs one after another. When all were dead, Indra began to weep and mourn. Then the gods ripped his pig-body open and he came out of it, and began to laugh, when he realised what a hideous dream he had—he, the king of the gods, to have become a pig, and to think that pig-life was the only life! Not only so, but to have wanted the whole universe to come into the pig-life.

The Purusha, when it identifies itself with nature, forgets that it is pure and infinite. The Purusha does not love, it is love itself. It does not exist, it is existence itself. The Soul does not know, it is knowledge itself. It is a mistake to say the Soul loves, exists, or knows. Love, existence, and knowledge are not the qualities of the Purusha, but its essence. When they get reflected upon something, you may call them the qualities of that something. They are not the qualities but the essence of the Purusha, the great Atman, the Infinite being, without birth or death, established in its own glory. It appears to have become so degenerate that if you approach to tell it, "You are not a pig," it begins to squeal and bite.

Thus is it with us all in this Maya, this dream world, where it is all misery, weeping and crying, where a few golden balls are rolled, and the world scrambles after them. You were never bound by laws, nature never had a bond for you. That is what the yogi tells you. Have patience to learn it. And the yogi shows how, by junction with nature, and identifying itself with the mind and the world, the Purusha thinks itself miserable. Then the yogi goes on to show you that the way out is through experience.

You have to get all this experience, but finish it quickly. We have placed ourselves in this net, and will have to get out. We have got ourselves caught in the trap, and we will have to work out our freedom. So get this experience of husbands, and wives and friends, and little loves; you will get through them safely if you never forget what you really are. Never forget this is only a momentary state, and that we have to pass through it.

Experience is the one great teacher—experience of

pleasure and pain—but know it is only experience. It leads, step by step, to that state where all things becomes small, and the Purusha so great that the whole universe seems as a drop in the ocean and falls off by its own nothingness. We have to go through different experiences, but let us never forget the ideal.

विशेषाविशेष-लिङ्गमात्रालिङ्गानि गुणपर्वाणि ॥19॥

The states of the qualities are the defined, the undefined, the indicated only, and the signless.

The system of yoga is built entirely on the philosophy of the Sankhyas, and here I shall remind you of the cosmology of the Sankhya philosophy.

According to the Sankhyas, nature is both the material and the efficient cause of the universe. In nature there are three sorts of materials, the Sattva, the Rajas, and the Tamas. The Tamas material is all that is dark, all that is ignorant and heavy. The Rajas is acitivity. The Sattva is calmness, light. Nature, before creation, is called by them Avyakta, undefined, or indiscrete; that is, in which there is no distinction of form or name, a state in which these three materials are held in perfect balance. Then the balance is disturbed, the three materials begin to mingle in various fashions, and the result is the universe.

In every man, also, these three material exist. When the Sattva material prevails, knowledge comes; when Rajas, activity; and when Tamas, darkness, lassitude, idleness and ignorance. According to the Sankhya theory, the highest manifestation of nature, consisting of the three materials, is what they call Mahat or intelligence, universal intelligence, of which each human intellect is a part.

In the Sankhya psychology there is a sharp distinction between Manas, the mind function, and the function of the Buddhi, intellect. The mind function is simply to collect and carry impressions and present them to the Buddhi, the individual Mahat, which determines upon it. Out of Mahat comes egoism, out of which again come the fine materials. The fine materials combine and become the gross material outside—the external universe.

The claim of the Sankhya philosophy is that beginning with the intellect down to a block of stone, all is the product of one substance, different only as finer to grosser states of experience. The finer is the cause, and the grosser is the effect. According to the Sankhya philosphy, beyond the whole of nature is the Purusha, which is not material at all. Purusha is not at all similar to anything else, either Buddhi, or mind, or the Tanmatras, or the gross materials. It is not akin to any one of these, it is entirely separate, entirely different in its nature, and from this they argue that the Purusha must be immortal, because it is not the result of combination. That which is not the result of combination cannot die. The Purushas or souls are infinite in number.

Now we shall understand the aphorism that the states of the qualities are defined, undefined, indicated only, and signless. By the "defined" are meant the gross elements, which we can sense. By the "undefined" are meant the very fine materials, the Tanmatras, which cannot be sensed by ordinary men. If you practise yoga, however, says Patanjali, after a while your perceptions will become so fine that you will actually see the Tanmatras. For instance, you have heard how every man has a certain light about him; every living being emits a certain light, and this, he says, can be seen by the yogi.

We do not all see it, but we all throw out these Tanmatras, just as flower continuously sends out fine particles which enable us to smell it. Every day of our lives we throw out a mass of good or evil, and everywhere we go to the atmosphere is full of these materials. That is how there came to the human mind, unconsciously, the idea of building temples and churches.

Why should man build churches in which to worship God? Why not worship him anywhere? Even if he did not know the reason, man found that the place where people worshipped God became full of good Tanmatras. Every day people go there, and the more they go, the holier they get, and the holier that place becomes. If any man who has not much Sattva in him goes there, the place will influence him and arouse his Sattva quality. Here, therefore, is the significance of all temples and holy places, but you must remember that their holiness depends on holy people congregating there.

The difficulty with man is that he forgets the original meaning, and puts the cart before the horse. It was men who made these places holy, and then the effect became the cause and made men holy. If the wicked only were to go there, it would become as bad as any other place. It is not the building, but the people that make a church, and that is what we always forget. That is why sages and holy persons, who have much of this Sattva quality, can send it out and exert a tremendous influence day and night on their surroundings. A man may become so pure that his purity will become tangible. Whosoever comes in contact with him becomes pure.

Next, "the indicated only" means the Buddhi, the intellect. "The indicated only" is the first manifestation of nature; from it all other manifestations proceed. The last is "the signless". There seems to be a great difference between modern science and all religions at this point. Every religion has the idea that the universe comes out of intelligence.

The theory of God, taking it in its psychological significance, apart from all ideas of personality, is that intelligence is first in the order of creation, and that out of intelligence comes what we call gross matter. Modern philosophers say that intelligence is the last to come. They say that unintelligent things slowly evolve into animals, and from animals into men. They claim that instead of everything coming out of intelligence, intelligence itself is the last to come. Both the religious and the scientific statement, though seeming directly opposed to each other are true.

Take an infinite series, A—B—A—B—A—B—, etc. The question is— which is first, A or B? If you take the series as A—B, you will say that A is the first, but if you take it as B—A, you will say that B is the first. It depends upon the way we look at it. Intelligence undergoes modification and becomes the gross matter, this again merges into intelligence, and thus the process goes on.

The Sankhyas, and other, religionists, put intelligence first, and the series becomes intelligence, then matter. The scientific man puts his finger on matter, and says matter, then intelligence. They both indicate the same chain. Indian philosophy, however, goes beyond both intelligence and matter, and finds a Purusha, or Self, which is beyond intelligence, of which intelligence is but the borrowed light.

द्रष्टा दृशिमात्रः शुद्धोऽपि प्रत्ययानुपश्यः ॥20॥

The seer is intelligence only, and though pure, sees through the colouring of the intellect.

This is, again, Sankhya philosophy. We have seen from the same philosophy that from the lowest form up to intelligence all is nature; beyond nature are Purushas (souls), which have no qualities. Then how does the soul appear to be happy or unhappy? By reflection. If a red flower is put near a piece of pure crystal, the crystal appears to be red, similarly, the appearances of happiness or unhappiness of the soul are but reflections.

The soul itself has no colouring. The soul is separate from nature. Nature is one thing, soul another, eternally separate. The Sankhyas say that intelligence is a compound, that it grows and wanes, that its changes, just as the body changes, and that it nature is nearly the same as that of the body.

As a finger-nail is to the body, so is body to intelligence. The nail is a part of the body, but it can be pared off hundreds of times, and the body will still last. Similarly, the intelligence lasts aeons, while this body can be "pared off", thrown off.

Yet intelligence cannot be immortal, because it changes—growing and waning. Anything that changes cannot be immortal. Certainly, intelligence is manufactured, and that very fact shows us that there must be something beyond that. It cannot be free, everything connected with matter is in nature, and, therefore, bound for ever.

Who is free? The free must certainly be beyond cause and effect. If you say that the idea of freedom is a delusion, I shall say that the idea of bondage is also a delusion. Two facts come into our consciousness, and stand or fall with each other. These are our notions of bondage and freedom. If we want to go through a wall, and our head bumps against that wall, we see we are limited by that wall. At the same time we find a will power, and think we can direct our will everywhere.

At every step these contradictory ideas come to us. We have to believe that we are free, yet at every moment we find we are not free. If one idea is a delusion, the other is also a delusion, and if one is true, the other also is true, because both stand upon the same basis—consciousness. The yogi says, both are true; that we are bound so far as intelligence goes, that we are free so far as the soul is concerned. It is the real nature of man, the soul, the Purusha, which is beyond all law of causation. Its freedom is percolating through layers of matter in various forms, intelligence, mind, etc. It is its light which is shining through all.

Intelligence has no light of its own. Each organ has a

particular centre in the brain; it is not that all the organs have one centre; each organ is separate. Why do all perceptions harmonise? Where do they get their unity? If it were in the brain, it would be necessary for all the organs, the eyes, the nose, the ears, etc., to have one centre only, while we know for certain that there are different centres for each. But a man can see and hear at the same time, so a unity must be there at the back of intelligence.

Intelligence is connected with the brain, but behind intelligence even stands the Purusha, the unit, where all different sensations and perceptions join and become one. The soul itself is the centre where all the different perceptions converge and become unified. That soul is free, and it is its freedom that tells you every moment that you are free. But you mistake, and mingle that freedom every moment with intelligence and mind.

You try to attribute that freedom to the intelligence and immediately find that intelligence is not free; you attribute that freedom to the body, and immediately nature tells you that you are again sense of freedom and bondage at the same time. The yogi analyses both what is free and what is bound, and his ignorance vanishes. He finds that the Purusha is free, is the essence of that knowledge which, coming through the Buddhi, becomes intelligence, and, as such, is bound.

तदर्थ एव दृश्यस्यात्मा ॥21॥

The nature of the experienced is for him.

Nature has no light of its own. As long as the Purusha is present in it, it appears as light. But the light is borrowed just as the moon's light is reflected. According to the yogis, all the manifestations of nature are caused by nature itself, but nature has no purpose in view, except to free the Purusha.

कृतार्थं प्रति नष्टमप्यनष्टं तदन्यसाधारणत्वात् ॥22॥

Though destroyed for him whose goal has been gained, yet it is not destroyed, being common to others.

The whole activity of nature is to make the soul know that it is entirely separate from nature. When the soul knows this, nature has no more attractions for it. But the whole of nature vanishes only for that man who has become free. There will always remain an infinite number of others, for whom nature will go on working.

स्वस्वामिशक्त्योः स्वरूपोपलब्धिहेतुः संयोगः ॥23॥

Junction is the cause of the realisation of the nature of both the powers, the experienced and its Lord.

According to this aphorism, both the powers of soul and nature become manifest when they are in conjunction. Then all manifestations are thrown out. Ignorance is the cause of this conjunction. We see every day that the cause of our pain or pleasure is always our joining ourselves with the body. If I were perfectly certain that I am not this body, I should take no notice of heat and cold, or anything of the kind.

This body is a combination. It is only a fiction to say that I have one body, you another, and the sun another. The whole universe is one ocean of matter, and you are the name of a little particle, and I of another, and the sun of another. We know that this matter is continuously changing. What is forming the sun one day, the next day may form the matter of our bodies.

तस्य हेतुरविद्या ॥24॥

Ignorance is its cause.

Through ignorance we have joined ourselves with a particular body, and thus opened ourselves to misery. This idea of body is a simple superstition. It is superstition that makes us happy or unhappy. It is superstition caused by ignorance that makes us feel heat and cold, pain and pleasure.

It is our business to rise above this superstition, and the yogi shows us how we can do this. It has been demonstrated that, under certain mental conditions, a man may be burned, yet he will feel no pain. The difficulty is that this sudden upheaval of the mind comes like a whirlwind one minute, and goes away the next. If, however, we gain it through yoga, we shall permanently attain to the separation of Self from the body.

तदभावात् संयोगाभावो हानं तद्दृशेः कैवल्यम् ॥25॥

There being absence of that (ignorance) there is absence of junction, which is the thing to be avoided; that is the independence of the seer.

According to yoga philosophy, it is through ignorance that the soul has been joined with nature. The aim is to get rid of nature's control over us. That is the goal of all religions. Each soul is potentially divine. The goal is to manifest this Divinity within, by controlling nature, external and internal. Do this either by work, or worship or psychic control, or philosophy—by one or more or all of these—and be free. This is the whole of religion.

Doctrines, or dogmas, or rituals, or books, or temples, or forms, are but secondary details. The yogi tries to reach this goal through psychic control. Until we can free ourselves from nature, we are slaves; as she dictates so we must go. The yogi claims that he who controls the mind controls matter also. The internal nature is much higher than the external and much more difficult to grapple with, much more difficult to control. Therefore he who has conquered the internal nature controls the whole universe; it becomes his servant.

Rajayoga propounds the methods of gaining this control. Forces higher than we know in physical nature will have to be subdued. This body is just the external crust of the mind. They are not two different things; they are just as the oyster and its shell. They are but two aspects of one thing; the internal substance of the oyster takes up matter from outside, and manufactures the shell.

In the same way the internal fine forces which are called mind, take up gross matter from outside, and from that manufactures this external shell, the body. If, then, we have control of the internal, it is very easy to have control of the external. Then again, these forces are not different. It is not that some forces are physical, and some mental; the physical forces are but the gross manifestations of the fine forces, just as the physical world is but the gross manifestation of the fine world.

विवेकख्यातिरविप्लवा हानोपायः ॥26॥

The means of destruction of ignorance is unbroken practice of discrimination.

This is the real goal of practice—discrimination between the real and the unreal, knowing that the Purusha is not nature, that it is neither matter nor mind, and that because it is not nature, it cannot possibly changes. It is only nature which changes, combining and re-combining, dissolving continually. When through constant practice we begin to discriminate, ignorance will vanish, and the Purusha will begin to shine in its real nature—omniscient, omnipotent, omnipresent.

तस्य सप्तधा प्रान्तभूमिः प्रज्ञा ॥27॥

His knowledge is of the sevenfold highest ground.

When this knowledge comes, it will come, as it were, in seven grades, one after the other; and when one of these begins, we know that we are getting knowledge. The first to appear will be that we have known what is to be known. The mind will cease to be dissatisfied. While we are aware of thirsting after knowledge, we begin to seek here and there, wherever we think we can get some truth, and failing to find it we become dissatisfied and seek in a fresh direction. All search is vain, until we begin to perceive that knowledge is within ourselves, that no one can help us, that we must help ourselves.

When we begin to practise the power of discrimination, the first sign that we are getting near truth will be that dissatisfied state will vanish. We shall feel quite sure that we have found the truth, and that it cannot be anything else but the truth. Then we may know that the sun is rising, that the morning is breaking for us, and taking courage, we must persevere until the goal is reached.

The second grade will be the absence of all pains. It will be impossible for anything in the universe, external or internal, to give us pain. The third will be the attainment of full knowledge. Omniscience will be ours. The forth will be the attainment of the end of all duty through discrimination.

Next will come what is called freedom of the Chitta. We shall realise that all difficulties and struggles, all vacillations of the mind, have fallen down, just as a stone rolls from the mountain top into the valley and never comes up again.

The next will be that the Chitta itself will realise that it melts away into its causes whenever we so desirc. Lastly, we shall find that we are established in our Self, that we have been alone throughout the universe, neither body nor mind was ever related, much less joined, to us. They were working their own way, and we, through ignorance, joined ourselves to them.

But we have been alone, omnipotent, omnipresent, ever blessed; our own Self was so pure and perfect that we required none else.

We required none else to make us happy, for we are happiness itself. We shall find that this knowledge does not depend on anything else; throughout the universe there can be nothing that will not become effulgent before our knowledge. This will be the last state, and the yogi will become peaceful and calm, never to feel any more pain, never to be again deluded, never to be touched by misery. He will know he is ever blessed, ever perfect, almighty.

योगाङ्गानुष्ठानादशुद्धिक्षये ज्ञानदीप्तिराविवेकख्यातेः ॥28॥

By the practice of the different parts of yoga the impurities being destroyed, knowledge becomes effulgent up to discrimination.

Now comes the practical knowledge. What we have just been speaking about is much higher. It is away above our heads, but is the ideal. It is first necessary to obtain physical and mental control. Then the realisation will become steady in that ideal. The ideal being known, what remains is to pracitse the method of reaching it.

यम-नियमासन-प्राणायाम-प्रत्याहार-धारणा-ध्यानसमाधयोऽष्टावङ्गानि ॥29॥

Yama, Niyama, Asana, Pranayama, Pratyahara, Dharana, Dhyana, and Samadhi are the eight limbs of yoga.

अहिंसा-सत्यास्तेय-ब्रह्मचर्यापरिग्रहा यमाः ॥30॥

Non-killing, truthfulness, non-stealing, continence, and non-receiving are called Yama.

A man who wants to be a perfect yogi must give up the sex idea. The soul has no sex; why should it degrade itself with sex ideas? Later on we shall understand better why these ideas must be given up. The mind of the man who receives gifts is acted on by the mind of the giver, so the receiver is likely to become degenerated. Receiving gifts is prone to destroy the independence of the mind, and make us slavish. Therefore, receive no gifts.

एते जाति-देश-काल-समयानवच्छिन्नाः सार्वभौमा महाव्रतम् ॥31॥

These, unbroken by time, place, purpose, and caste rules, are (universal) great vows.

These practices—non-killing, truthfulness, non-stealing, chastity, and non-receiving—are to be practised by every man, woman, and child; by every soul, irrespective of nation, country, or position.

शौच-सन्तोष-तपः स्वाध्यायेश्वरप्रणिधानानि नियमाः ॥32॥

Internal and external purification, contentment, mortification, study, and worship of God are the Niyamas.

External purification is keeping the body pure; a dirty man will never be a yogi. There must be internal purification also. That is obtained by the virtues named in I.33. Of course, internal purity is of greater value than external, but both are necessary, and external purity, without internal, is of no good.

वितर्कबाधने प्रतिपक्षभावनम् ॥33॥

To obstruct thoughts which are inimical to yoga, contrary thoughts should be brought.

That is the way to practise the virtues that have been stated. For instance, when a big wave of anger has come into the mind, how are we to control that? Just by raising an opposing wave. Think of love. Sometimes a mother is very angry with her husband, and while in that state, the baby come in, and she kisses the baby; the old wave dies out and a new wave arises, love for the child. That suppresses the other one. Love is opposite to anger. Similarly, when the idea of stealing comes, non-stealing should be thought of; when the idea of receiving gifts comes, replace it by a contrary thought.

वितर्का हिंसादयः कृतकारितानुमोदिता लोभक्रोध- मोहपूर्वका मृदुमध्याधिमात्रा दुःखाज्ञानानन्तफला इति प्रतिपक्षभावनम् ॥34॥

The obstructions to yoga are killing, falsehood, etc., whether committed, caused, or approved; either through avarice, or anger, or ignorance; whether slight, middling, or great; and they result in infinite ignorance and misery. This is (the method of) thinking the contrary.

It I tell a lie, or cause another to tell one, or approve of another doing so, it is equally sinful. If it is a very mild lie, still it is a lie. Every vicious thought will rebound, every thought of hatred which you may have thought in a cave even is stored up, and will one day come back to you with tremendous power in the form of some misery here. If you project hatred and jealousy, they will rebound on you with compound interest. No power can avert them; when once you have put them in motion, you will have to bear them. Remembering this will prevent you from doing wicked things.

अहिंसाप्रतिष्ठायां तत्सन्निधौ वैरत्यागः ॥35॥

Non-killing being established, in his presence all enmities cease (in others).

If a man gets the ideal of non-injuring others before him even animals which are by their nature ferocious will become peaceful. The tiger and the lamb will play together before that yogi. When you have come to that state, then alone you will understand that you have become firmly established in non-injuring.

सत्यप्रतिष्ठायां क्रियाफलाश्रयत्वम् ॥36॥

By the establishment of truthfulness the yogi gets the power of gaining for himself and others the fruits of work without the works.

When this power of truth will be established with you, then even in dream you will never tell an untruth. You will be true in thought, word, and deed. Whatever you say will be truth. You may say to a man, "Be blessed," and that man will be blessed. If a man is diseased, and you say to him, "Be thou cured," he will be cured immediately.

अस्तेयप्रतिष्ठायां सर्वरत्नोपस्थानम् ॥37॥

By the establishment of non-stealing all wealth comes to the yogi.

The more you fly from nature, the more she follows you; and if you do not care for her at all, she becomes your slave.

ब्रह्मचर्यप्रतिष्ठायां वीर्यलाभः ॥38॥

By the establishment of continence energy is gained.

The chaste brain has tremendous energy and gigantic will-power. Without chastity there can be no spiritual strength. Continence gives wonderful control over mankind. The spiritual leaders of men have been very continent, and this is what gave them power. Therefore, the yogi must be continent.

अपरिग्रहस्थैर्ये जन्मकथन्तासंबोधः ॥39॥

When he is fixed in non-receiving, he gets the memory of past life.

When a man does not receive presents, he does not become beholden to others, but remains independent and free. His mind becomes pure. With every gift, he is likely to receive the evils of the giver. If he does not receive, the mind is purified, and the first power it gets is memory of past life. Then alone the yogi becomes perfectly fixed in his ideal. He sees that he has been coming and going many times, so he becomes determined that this time he will be free, that he will no more come and go, and be the slave of Nature.

शौचात्स्वाङ्गजुगुप्सा परैरसंसर्गः ॥40॥

Internal and external cleanliness being established, arises disgust for one's own body, and non-intercourse with others.

When there is real purification of the body, external and internal, there arises neglect of the body, and the ideal of keeping it nice vanishes. A face which others call most beautiful will appear to the yogi as merely animal, if there is no intelligence behind it. What the world call a very common face he regards as heavenly, if the spirit shines behind it. This thirst after body is the great bane of human life. So the first sign of the establishment of purity is that you do not care to think you are a body. It is only when purity comes that we get rid of the body idea.

सत्त्वशुद्धि-सौमनस्यैकाग्र्येन्द्रियजयात्मदर्शनयोग्यत्वानि च ॥41॥

There also arises purification of the Sattva, cheerfulness of the mind, concentration, conquest of the organs, and fitness for the realisation of the Self.

By the practice of cleanliness, the Sattva material prevails and the mind becomes concentrated and cheerful. The first sign that you are becoming religious is that you are becoming cheerful. When a man is gloomy, that may be dyspepsia, but it is not religion. A pleasurable feeling is the nature of the Sattva. Everything is pleasurable to the Sattvika man, and when this comes, know that you are progressing in yoga. All pain is caused by Tamas, so you must get rid of that; moroseness is one of the results of Tamas.

The strong, the well-knit, the young, the healthy, the daring alone are fit to be yogis. To the yogi everything is bliss, every human face that he sees brings cheerfulness to him. That is the sign of a virtuous man. Misery is caused by sin, and by no other cause. What business have you with clouded faces? It is terrible. If you have a clouded face, do not go out that day, shut yourself up in your room. What right have you to carry this disease out into the world? When your mind has become controlled, you have control over the whole body; instead of being a slave to this machine, the machine is your slave. Instead of this machine being able to drag the soul down. it becomes its greatest helpmate.

सन्तोषादनुत्तमः सुखलाभः ॥42॥

From contentment comes supcrlative huppiness.

कायेन्द्रियसिद्धिरशुद्धिक्षयात्तपसः ॥43॥

The result of mortification is bringing powers to the organs and the body, by destroying the impurity.

The results of mortification are seen immediately, sometimes by heightened power of vision, hearing things at a distance, and so on.

स्वाध्यायादिष्टदेवतासम्प्रयोगः ॥44॥

By the repetition of the Mantra comes the realisation of the intended deity.

The higher the beings that you want to get the harder is the practice.

समाधिसिद्धिरीश्वरप्रणिधानात् ॥45॥

By sacrificing all to Ishvara comes Samadhi.

By resignation to the Lord, Samadhi becomes perfect.

स्थिरसुखमासनम् ॥46॥

Posture is that which is firm and pleasant.

Now comes Asana, posture. Until you can get a firm seat

you cannot practise the breathing and other exercises. Firmness of seat means that you do not feel the body at all. In the ordinary way, you will find that as soon as you sit for a few minutes all sorts of disturbance come into the body; but when you have got beyond the idea of a concrete body, you will lose all sense of the body. You will feel neither pleasure not pain. And when you take your body up again, it will feel so rested. It is the only perfect rest that you can give to the body. When you have succeeded in conquering the body and keeping it firm, your practice will remain firm, but while you are disturbed by the body, your nerves become disturbed, and you cannot concentrate the mind.

प्रयत्नशैथिल्यानन्तसमापत्तिभ्याम् ॥47॥

By lessening the natural tendency (for restlessness) and meditating on the unlimited, posture becomes firm and pleasant.

We can make the seat firm by thinking of the infinite. We cannot think of the Absolute infinite, but we can think of the infinite sky.

ततो द्वन्द्वानभिघातः ॥48॥

Seat being conquered, the dualities do not obstruct.

The dualities, good and bad, heat and cold, and all the pairs of opposite, will not then disturb you.

तस्मिन् सति श्वासप्रश्वासयोर्गतिविच्छेदः प्राणायामः ॥49॥

Controlling the motion of the exhalation and the inhalation follows after this.

When posture has been conquered, then the motion of the Prana is to be broken and controlled. Thus we come to Pranayama, the controlling of the vital forces of the body. **Prana is not breath, though it is usually so translated. It is the sum total of the cosmic energy. It is the energy that is in each body, and its most apparent manifestation is the**

motion of the lungs. This motion is caused by Prana drawing in the breath, and it is what we seek to control in Pranayama. We begin by controlling the breath, as the easiest way of getting control of the Prana.

बाह्याभ्यन्तरस्तम्भवृत्तिः देशकालसंख्याभिः परिदृष्टो दीर्घ सूक्ष्मः ॥50॥

Its modifications are either external or internal, or motionless, regulated by place, time, and number, either long or short.

The three sorts of motion of Pranayama are, one by which we draw the breath in , another by which we throw it out, and the third action is when the breath is held in the lungs, or stopped from entering the lungs. These, again, are varied by place and time. By place is meant that the Prana is held to some particular part of the body. By time is meant how long the Prana should be confined to ascertain place, and so we are told how many seconds to keep one motion, and how many seconds to keep another. The result of this Pranayama is Udghata, awakening the Kundalini.

बाह्याभ्यान्तरविषयाक्षेपी चतुर्थः ॥51॥

The fourth is restraining the Prana by reflecting on external or internal object.

This is the fourth sort of Pranayama, in which the Kumbhaka is brought about by long practice attended with reflection, which is absent in the other three.

ततः क्षीयते प्रकाशावरणम् ॥52॥

From that, the covering to the light of the Chitta is attenuated.

The Chitta has, by its own nature, all knowledge. It is made of Sattva particles, but is covered by Rajas and Tamas particles, and by Pranayama this covering is removed.

धारणासु च योग्यता मनसः ॥53॥

The mind becomes fit for Dharana.

After this covering has been removed. We are able to concentrate the mind.

स्वविषयासम्प्रयोगे चित्तस्वरूपानुकार इवेन्द्रियाणां प्रत्याहारः ॥54॥

The drawing in of the organs is by their giving up their own objects and taking the form of the mind-stuff, as it were.

The organs are separate states of the mind-stuff. I see a book; the form is not in the book, it is in the mind. Something is outside which calls that form up. The real form is in the Chitta. The organs identify themselves with, and take the forms of, whatever comes to them. If you can restrain the mind-stuff from taking these forms, the mind will remain calm. This is called Pratyahara.

ततः परमा वश्यतेन्द्रियाणाम् ॥55॥

Thence arises supreme control of the organs.

When the yogi has succeeded in preventing the organs from taking the forms of external objects, and in making them remain one with the mind-stuff, then comes perfect control of the organs. When the organs are perfectly under control, every muscle and nerve will be under control, because the organs are the centres of all the sensations, and of all actions.

These organs are divided into organs of work and organs of sensation. When the organs are controlled, the yogi can control all feeling and doing; Then alone one begins to feel joy in being born; then one can truthfully say, "Blessed am I that I was born." When that control of the organs is obtained, we feel how wonderful this body really is.

3

The Powers Attained by Yoga

We have now come to the chapter in which the yoga powers are described.

देशबन्धश्चित्तस्य धारणा ॥1॥

Dharana is holding the mind on to some particular object.

Dharana (concentration) is when the mind holds on to some objects, either in the body or outside the body, and keeps itself in that state.

तत्र प्रत्ययैकतानता ध्यानम् ॥2॥

An unbroken flow of knowledge in that object is Dhyana.

The mind tries to think of one object, to hold itself to one particular spot, as the top of the head, the heart, etc., and if the mind succeeds in receiving the sensations only through that part of the body, and through no other part, that would be Dharana, and when the mind succeeds in keeping itself in that state for some time, it is called Dhyana (meditation).

तदेवार्थमात्रनिर्भासं स्वरूपशून्यमिव समाधिः ॥3॥

When that, giving up all forms, reflects only the meaning, it is Samadhi.

That comes when in meditation the form or the external part is given up. Suppose I were meditating on a book, and that I have gradually succeeded in concentrating the mind on it, and perceiving only the internal sensations, the meaning unexpressed in any form—that state of Dhyana is called Samadhi.

त्रयमेकत्र संयमः ॥4॥

(These) three (when practised) in regard to one object is Samyama.

When a man can direct his mind to any particular objects and fix it there, and then keep it there for a long time, separating the objects from the internal part, this is Samyama; or Dharana, Dhyana and Samadhi, one following the other, and making one. The form of the thing has vanished, and only its meaning remains in the mind.

तज्जयात् प्रज्ञाऽऽलोकः ॥5॥

By the conquest of that comes light of knowledge.

When one has succeeded in making this Samyama, all powers come under his control. This is the great instrument of the yogi. The objects of knowledge are infinite, and they are divided into the gross, grosser, grossest and the fine, finer, finest and so on. This Samyama should be first applied to gross things, and when you begin to get knowledge of this gross, slowly, by stages, it should be brought to finer things.

तस्य भूमिषु विनियोगः ॥6॥

That should be employed in stages.

This is a note of warning not to attempt to go too fast.

त्रयमन्तरङ्गं पूर्वेभ्यः ॥7॥

These three are more internal than those that precede.

Before these we had the Pratyahara, the Pranayama, the Asana, the Yama and Niyama; they are external parts of the three—Dharana, Dhyana and Samadhi. When a man has attained to them, he may attain to omniscience and omnipotence, but that would not be salvation. These three would not make the mind Nirvikalpa, changeless, but would leave the seeds for getting bodies again. Only when the seeds are, as the yogi says, "fried," do they lose the possibility of producing further plants. These powers cannot fry the seed.

तदपि बहिरङ्गं निर्बीजस्य ॥8॥

But even they are external to the seedless (Samadhi).

Compared with that seedless Samadhi, therefore, even these are external. We have not yet reached the real Samadhi, the highest, but a lower stage, in which this universe still exists as we see it, and in which are all these powers.

व्युत्थान-निरोधसंस्कारयोरभिभव-प्रादुर्भावौ निरोधक्षणचित्तान्वयो निरोध-परिणामः ॥9॥

By the suppression of the disturbed impressions of the mind, and by the rise of impressions of control, the mind which persists in that moment of control, is said to attain the controlling modifications.

That is to say, in this first state of Samadhi the modifications of the mind have been controlled, but not perfectly, because if they were, there would be no modifications. If there is a modification which impels the mind to rush out through the senses, and the yogi tries to control it, that very control itself will be a modification. One wave will be checked by another wave, so it will not be real Samadhi in which all the waves subside, as control itself will be a wave. Yet this lower Samadhi is very much nearer to the higher Samadhi than when the mind comes bubbling out.

तस्य प्रशान्तवाहिता संस्कारात् ॥10॥

Its flow becomes steady by habit.

The flow of this continuous control of the mind becomes steady when practised day after day, and the mind obtains the faculty of constant concentration.

सर्वार्थतैकाग्रतयोः क्षयोदयौ चित्तस्य समाधि परिणामः ॥11॥

Taking in all sorts of objects, and concentrating upon one object, these two powers being destroyed and manifested respectively, the Chitta gets the modification called Samadhi.

The mind takes up various objects, runs into all sorts of things. That is the lower state, There is a higher state of the mind, when it takes up one object and excludes all others, of which Samadhi is the result.

शान्तोदितौ तुल्यप्रत्ययौ चित्तस्यैकाग्रता-परिणामः ॥12॥

The one-pointedness of the Chitta is when the impression that is past and that which is present are similar.

How are we to know that the mind has become concentrated? Because the idea of time will vanish. The more time passes unnoticed the more concentrated we are. In common life we see that when we are interested in a book we do not note the time at all; and when we have the book, we are often surprised to find how many hours have passed. All time will have the tendency to come and stand in the one present. So the definition is given: When the past and present come and stand in one, the mind is said to be concentrated.

एतेन भतेन्द्रियेषु धर्मलक्षणावस्थापरिणामा व्याख्याताः ॥13॥

By this is explained the threefold transformation of form, time and state, in fine or gross matter and in the organs.

By the threefold changes in the mind-stuff as to form,

time and state are explained the corresponding changes in gross and subtle matter and in the organs. Suppose there is a lump of gold. It is transformed into a bracelet and again into an earring. These are changes as to form. The same phenomena looked at from the standpoint of time give us change as to time. Again the bracelet or the earring may be bright or dull, thick or thin, and so on. This is change as to state.

Now referring to the aphorisms 9, 11, and 12, the mind-stuff is changing into Vrittis—this is change as to form. That it passes through past, present and future moments of time is change as to time. That the impressions vary as to intensity within one particular period, say, present, is change as to state. The concentrations taught in the preceding aphorisms were to give the yogi voluntary control over the transformations of his mind-stuff, which alone will enable him to make the Samyama named in III. 4.

शान्तोदिताव्यपदेश्यधर्मानुपातो धर्मी ॥14॥

That which is acted upon by transfor-mations, either past, present, or yet to be manifested is the qualified.

That is to say, the qualified is the substance which is being acted upon by time and by the Samskaras, and getting changed and being manifested always.

क्रमान्यत्वं परिणामान्यत्वे हेतुः ॥15॥

The succession of changes is the cause of manifold evolution.

परिणामत्रयसंयमादतीतानागतज्ञानम् ॥16॥

By making Samyama on the three sorts of changes comes the knowledge of past and future.

We must not lose sight of the first definition of Samyama. When the mind has attained to that state when it identifies itself with the internal impression of the objects, leaving the external, and when, by long practice, that is retained by the mind and the mind can get into that state in a moment, that is Samyama. If a man in that state wants to know the past and future, he has to make a Samyama on the changes in the Samskaras (III. 13). Some are working now at present, some have worked out, and some are waiting to work. So by making a Samyama on these he knows the past and future.

शब्दार्थप्रत्ययानामितरेतराध्यासात्सङ्करस्तत्प्रविभागसंयमात् सर्वभूतरुतज्ञानम् ॥17॥

By making Samyama on word, meaning and knowledge, which are ordinarily confused, comes the knowledge of all animal sounds.

The word represents the external cause, the meaning represents the internal vibration that travels to the brain through the channels of the Indriyas, conveying the external impression to the mind, and knowledge represents the reaction of the mind, with which comes perception. These three, confused, make our sense objects.

Suppose I hear a word; there is first the external vibration, next the internal sensation carried to the mind by the organ of hearing, then the mind reacts, and I know the word. The word I know is a mixture of the three— vibration, sensation, and reaction. Ordinarily these three are inseparable; but by practice the yogi can separate them. When a man has attained to this, if he makes a Samyama on any sound, he understands the meaning which that sound was intended to express, whether it was made by man or by any other animal.

संस्कारसाक्षात्करणात् पूर्वजातिज्ञानम् ॥18॥

By perceiving the impressions, (comes) the knowledge of past life.

Each experience that we have, comes in the form of a wave in the Chitta, and this subsides and becomes finer and finer, but is never lost. It remains there in minute form, and if we can bring this wave up again, it becomes memory. So, if the yogi can make a Samyama on these past impressions in the mind, he will begin to remember all his past lives.

प्रत्ययस्य परिचित्तज्ञानम् ॥19॥

By making Samyama on the signs in another's body, knowledge of his mind comes.

Each man has particular signs on his body, which differentiate him from other; when the yogi makes a Samyama on these signs he knows the nature of that mind of the person.

न च तत् सालम्बनं तस्याविषयीभूतत्वात् ॥20॥

But not its contents, that not being the objects of theSamyama.

He would not know the contents of the mind by making a Samyama on the body. There would be required a twofold Samyama, first on the signs in the body, and then on the mind itself. The yogi would then know everything that is in that mind.

कायरूपसंयमात्तद्ग्राह्यशक्ति-स्तम्भे चक्षुःप्रकाशासंयोगेऽन्तर्धानम् ॥21॥

By making Samyama on the form of the body, the perceptibility of the form being obstructed and the power of manifestation in the eye being separated, the yogis's body becomes unseen.

A yogi standing in the midst of this room can apparently vanish. He does not really vanish, but he will not be seen by anyone. The form and the body are, as it were, separated. You must remember that this can only be done when the yogi has attained to that power of concentration when form and the thing formed have been separated. Then he makes a Samyama on that, and the power to perceive forms is obstructed, because the power of perceiving forms comes from the junction of form and thing formed.

एतेन शब्दाद्यन्तर्धानमुक्तम् ॥22॥

By this the disappearance or concealment of words which are being spoken and such other things are also explained.

सोपक्रमं निरुपक्रमं च कर्म तत्संयमादपरान्तज्ञानमरिष्टेभ्यो वा ॥23॥

Karma is of two kinds—soon to be fructified and late to be fructified. By making Samyama on these, or by the signs called Arishta, portents, the yogi knows the exact time of separation from their bodies.

When a yogi makes a Samyama on his own Karma, upon those impressions in his mind which are now working, and those which are just waiting to work, he knows exactly by those that are waiting when his body will fall. He knows when he will die, at what hour, even at what minute. The Hindus think very much of that knowledge or consciousness of the nearness of death, because it is taught in the Gita that the thoughts at the moment of departure are great powers in determining the next life.

मैत्र्यादिषु बलानि ॥24॥

By making Samyama on friendship mercy, etc. (I.33), the yogi excels in the respective qualities.

बलेषु हस्तिबलादीनि ॥25॥

By making Samyama on the strength of the elephant and others, their respective strength comes to the yogi.

When a yogi has attained to this Samyama and wants

strength, he makes a Samyama on the strength of the elephant and gets it. Infinite energy is at the disposal of everyone if he only knows how to get it. The yogi has discovered the science of getting it.

प्रवृत्यालोकन्यासात् सूक्ष्म-व्यवहित-विप्रकृष्टज्ञानम् ॥26॥

By making Samyama on the effulgent light (I.36), comes the knowledge of the fine, the obstructed, and the remote.

When the yogi makes Samyama on that Effulgent Light in the heart. he sees things which are very remote, things, for instance, that are happening in a distant place, and which are obstructed by mountain barriers, and also things which are very fine.

भुवनज्ञानं सूय संयमात् ॥27॥

By making Samyama on the sun, (comes) the knowledge of the world.

चन्द्रेताराव्यूहज्ञानम् ॥28॥

On the moon, (comes) the knowledge of the cluster of stars.

ध्रुवेतद्गतिज्ञानम् ॥29॥

On the pole-star, (comes) the knowledge of the motions of the stars.

नाभिचक्रेकायव्यूहज्ञानम् ॥30॥

On the navel circle, (comes) the knowledge of the constitution of the body.

कण्ठकूपेक्षुतिपपासानिवृत्तिः ॥31॥

On the hollow of the throat, (comes) cessation of hunger.

When a man is very hungry, if he can make Samyama on the hollow of the throat, hunger ceases.

कूर्मनाड्यां स्थैर्यम् ॥32॥

On the nerve called Kurma, (comes) fixity of the body.

When he is practising, the body is not disturbed.

मूर्धज्योतिषि सिद्धदर्शनम् ॥33॥

On the light emanating from the top of the head, sight of the Siddhas.

The Siddhas are beings who are a little above ghosts. When the yogi concentrates his mind on the top of his head, he will see these Siddhas. The word Siddha does not refer to those men who have become free—a sense in which it is often used.

प्रातिभाद्वा सर्वम् ॥34॥

Or by the power of Pratibha, all knowledge.

All these can come without any Samyama to the man who has the power of Pratibha (spontaneous enlightement from purity). When a man has risen to a high state of Pratibha, he has the great light. All things are apparent to him. Everything comes to him naturally without making Samyama.

हृदये चित्त-संवित् ॥35॥

In the heart, knowledge of minds.

Enjoyment comes from the non-discrimination of the soul and Sattva which are totally different because the latter's actions are for another. Samyama on the self-centred one gives knowledge of the Purusha.

All action of Sattva, a modification of Prakriti characterised by light and happiness, is for the soul. When Sattva is free from egoism and illuminated with the pure intelligence of Purusha, it is called the self-centred one, because in that state it becomes independent of all relations.

ततः प्रातिभश्रावणवेदनादर्शास्वादवार्ता जायन्ते ॥37॥

From that arises the knowledge belonging to Pratibha and (supernatural) hearing, touching, seeing, tasting and smelling.

ते समाधावुपसर्गा व्युत्थाने सिद्धयः ॥38॥

These are obstacles to Samadhi; but they are powers in the worldly state.

To the yogi knowledge of the enjoyments of the world comes by the junction of the Purusha and the mind. If he wants to make Samyama on the knowledge that they are two different things, nature and soul, he gets knowledge of the Purusha. From that arises discrimination. When he has got that discrimination, he gets the Pratibha, the light of supreme genius.

These powers, however, are obstructions to the attainment of the highest goal, the knowledge of the pure Self, and freedom. These are, as it were, to be met in the way; and if the yogi rejects them, he attains the highest. If he is tempted to acquire these, his further progress is barred.

बन्धकारणशैथिल्यात् प्रचारसंवेदनाच्च चित्तस्य परशरीरावेशः ॥39॥

When the cause of bondage of the Chitta has become loosened the yogi, by his knowledge of its channels of activity (the nerves), enters another's body.

The yogi can enter a dead body and make it get up and move, even while he himself is working in another body. Or he can enter a living body and hold that man's mind and organs in check, and for the time being act through the body of that man. That is done by the yogi coming to this discrimination of Purusha and nature. If he wants to enter another's body, he makes a Samyama on that body and enters it, because, not only is his soul omnipresent, but his mind also, as the yogi teaches. It is one bit of the universal mind. Now, however, it can only work through the nerve currents in this body, but when the yogi has loosened himself from these nerve currents, he can work through other things.

उदानजयाज्जलपङ्ककण्टकादिष्वसङ्ग उत्क्रान्तिश्च ॥40॥

By conquering the current called Udana, the yogi does not sink in water or in swamps, he can walk on thorns etc., and can die at will.

Udana is the name of the nerve current that governs the lungs and all the upper parts of the body, and when he is master of it, he becomes light in weight. He does not sink in water: he can walk on thorns and sword blades, and stand in fire, and can depart this life whenever he likes.

समानजयात् प्रज्वलनम् ॥41॥

By the conquest of the current Samana he is surrounded by a blaze of light.

Whenever he likes, light flashes from his body.

श्रोत्राकाशयोः सम्बन्धसंयमाद्दिव्यं श्रोत्रम् ॥42॥

By making Samyama on the relation between the ear and the Akasha comes divine hearing.

There is the Akasha, the ether, and the instrument, the ear. By making Samyama on them the yogi gets supernormal hearing: he hears everything. Anything spoken or sounded miles away he can hear.

कायाकाशयोः सम्बन्धसंयमाल्लघुतूलसमापत्तेश्चाकाशगमनम् ॥43॥

By making Samyama on the relation between the

Akasha and the body and becoming light as cotton-wool etc., through meditation on them, the yogi goes through the skies.

This Akasha is the material of this body: it is only Akasha in a certain form that has become the body. If the yogi makes a Samyama on this Akasha material of his body, it acquires the lightness of Akasha, and he can go anywhere through the air. So in the other case also.

बहिरकल्पिता वृत्तिर्महाविदेहा ततः प्रकाशावरणक्षयः ॥44॥

By making Samyama on the "real modifications" of the mind, outside of the body, called great disembodiedness, comes disappearance of the covering to light.

The mind in its foolishness thinks that it is working in this body. Why should I be bound by one system of nerves, and put the ego only in the body, if the mind is omnipresent? There is no reason why I should. The yogi wants to feel the ego wherever he likes. The mental waves which arise in the absence of egoism in the body are called "real modifications" or "great disembodiedness". When he has succeeded in making Samyama on these modifications, all covering to light goes away, and all darkness and ignorance vanish. Everything appears to him to be full of knowledge.

स्थूल-स्वरूप-सूक्ष्मान्वयार्थवत्वसंयमाद्भूतजयः ॥45॥

By making Samyama on the gross and fine forms of the elements, their essential traits, the inherence of the Gunas in them and on their contributing to the experience of the soul, comes mastery of the elements.

The yogi makes Samyama on the elements first on the gross, and then on the finer states. This Samyama is taken up more by a sect of the Buddhists. They take a lump of clay and make Samyama on that, and gradually they begin to see the fine materials of which it is composed, and when they have known all the fine materials in it, they get power over that element. So with all the elements. The yogi can conquer them all.

ततोऽणिमादिप्रादुर्भावः कायसम्पत्तद्धर्मानभिघातश्च ॥46॥

From that comes minuteness and the rest of the powers, "glorification of the body", and indestructibleness of the bodily qualities.

This means that the yogi has attained the eight powers. He can make himself as minute as a particle, or as huge as a mountain, as heavy as the earth, or as light as the air, he can reach anything he likes, he can rule everything he wants, he can conquer everything he wants and so on. A lion will sit at his feet like a lamb, and all his desires will be fulfilled at will.

रूप-लावण्य-बल-वज्रसंहननत्वानि कायसम्पत् ॥47॥

The "glorification of the body" is beauty, complexion, strength, adamantine hardness.

The body becomes indestructible. Nothing can injure it. Nothing can destroy it until the yogi wishes. "Breaking the rod of time he lives in this universe with his body." In the Vedas it is written that for that man there is no more disease, death or pain.

ग्रहण-स्वरूपास्मितान्वयार्थवत्वसंयमादिन्द्रियजयः ॥48॥

By making Samyama on the objectivity and power of illumination of the organs, on egoism, the inherence of the Gunas in them and on their contributing to the experience of the soul, comes the conquest of the organs.

In the perception of external objects the organs leave

their place in the mind and go towards the object: this is followed by knowledge. Egoism also is present in the act. When the yogi makes Samyama on these and the other two by gradation, he conquers the organs. Take up anything that you see or feel, a book for instance; first concentrate the mind on it, then on the knowledge that is in the form of a book, and then on the ego that sees the book, and so on. By that practice all the organs will be conquered.

ततो मनोजवित्वं विकरणभावः प्रधानजयश्च ॥49॥

From that comes to the body the power of rapid movement like the mind, power of the organs independently of the body, and conquest of nature.

Just as by the conquest of the elements comes glorified body, so from the conquest of the organs will come the above-mentioned powers.

सत्त्वपुरुषान्यताख्यातिमात्रस्य सर्वभावाधिष्ठातृत्वं सर्वज्ञातृत्वञ्च ॥50॥

By making Samyama on the discrimination between the Sattva and Purusha come omnipotence and omniscience.

When nature has been conquered, and the difference between the Purusha and nature realised—that the Purusha is indestructible, pure and perfect—then come omnipotence and omniscience.

तद्वैराग्यादपि दोषबीजक्षये कैवल्यम् ॥51॥

By giving up even these powers comes the destruction of the very seed of evil, which leads of Kaivalya.

He attains aloneness, independence, and becomes free. When one gives up even the ideas of omnipotence and omniscience, there comes entire rejection of enjoyment, of the temptations from celestial beings. When the yogi has seen all these wonderful powers, and rejected them, he reaches the goal. What are all these powers? Simply manifestations. They are no better than dreams. Even omnipotence is a dream. It depends on the mind. So long as there is a mind it can be understood, but the goal is beyond even the mind.

स्थान्युपनिमन्त्रणे सङ्गस्मयाकरणं पुनरनिष्टप्रसङ्गात् ॥52॥

The yogi should not feel allured or flattered by overtures of celestial beings for fear of evil again.

There are other dangers too; gods and other beings come to tempt the yogi. They do not want anyone to be perfectly free. They are jealous, just as we are, and worse than us sometimes. They are very much afraid of losing their places. Those yogis who do not reach perfection die and become gods; leaving the direct road they go into one of the side-streets and get these powers. Then, again, they have to be born. But he who is strong enough to withstand these temptations and go straight to the goal, becomes free.

क्षण-तत्क्रमयोः संयमाद्विवेकजं ज्ञानम् ॥53॥

By making Samyama on a particle of time and its precession and succession comes discrimination.

How are we to avoid all these things, these Devas, and heavens, and powers? By discrimination, by knowing good from evil. Therefore, a Samyama is given by which the power of discrimination can be strengthened. This is by making a Samyama on a particle of time, and the time preceding and following it.

जाति-लक्षण-देशैरन्यताऽनवच्छेदात्तुल्ययोस्ततः प्रतिपत्तिः ॥54॥

Those things which cannot be differentiated by species, signs, and place, even they will be discriminated by the above Samyama.

The misery that we suffer comes form ignorance, from non-discrimination between the real and the unreal. We all take the bad for the good, the dream for the reality. Soul is the only reality, and we have forgotten it. Body is an unreal dream, and we think we are all bodies. This non-discrimination is the cause of misery. It is caused by ignorance. When discrimination comes, it brings strength, and then alone can we avoid all these various idea of body, heavens, and gods.

This ignorance arises through differentiating by species, sign and place. For instance, take a cow. The cow is differentiated from the dog by species. Even with the cows alone how do we make the distinction between one cow and another? By signs. If two objects are exactly similar, they can be distinguished if they are in different places. When objects are so mixed up that even these differences will not help us, the power of discrimination acquired by the above-mentioned practice will give us the ability to distinguish them.

The highest philosophy of the yogi is based upon this fact, that the Purusha is pure and perfect, and is the only "simple" that exists in this universe. The body and mind are compounds, and yet we are ever identifying ourselves with them. This is the great mistake that the distinction has been attained, man sees that everything in this world, mental and physical, is a compound, and, as such, cannot be the Purusha.

तारकं सर्वविषयं सर्वथाविषयमक्रमञ्चेति विवेकजं ज्ञानम् ॥55॥

The saving knowledge is that knowledge of discrimination which simultaneously cover all objects, in all their variations.

Saving because the knowledge takes the yogi across the ocean of birth and death. The whole of Prakriti in all its states, subtle and gross, is within the grapes of this knowledge. There is no succession in perception by this knowledge; it takes in all things simultaneously, at a glance.

सत्त्वपुरुषयोः शुद्धिसाम्ये कैवल्यमिति ॥56॥

By the similarity of purity between the Sattva and Purusha comes Kaivalya.

When the soul realises that it depends on nothing in the universe, from gods to the lowest atom, that is called Kaivalya (isolation) and perfection. It is attained when this mixture of purity and impurity called Sattva (intellect) has been made as pure as the Purusha itself; then the Sattva reflects only the unqualified essence of purity, which is the Purusha.

4

Independence

जन्मौषधि-मन्त्र-तपः-समाधिजाः सिद्धयः ॥1॥

The Siddhis (powers) are attained by birth, chemical means, power of word, mortification, or concentration.

Sometimes a man is born with the Siddhis, powers of course, those he had earned in his previous incarnation. This time he is born, as it were, to enjoy the fruits of them. It is said of Kapila, the great father of the Sankhya philosophy, that he was a born Siddha, which means literally a man who has attained to success.

The yogis claim that these powers can be gained be chemical means. All of you know that chemistry originally began as alchemy; men went in search of the philosopher's stone and elixirs of life, and so forth. In India there was a sect called the Rasayanas. Their idea was that ideality, knowledge, spirituality, and religion were all very right, but that the body was the only instrument by which to attain to all these. If the body came to an end every now and again , it would take so much more time to attain to the goal.

For instance, a man wants to practise yoga, or wants to become spiritual. Before he has advanced very far he dies. Then he takes another body and begins again, then dies, and so on. In this way much time will be lost in dying and being born again. If the body could be made strong and perfect, so that it would get rid of birth and death, we should have so much more time to become spiritual. So these Rasayanas say, first make the body very strong.

They claim that this body can be made immortal. Their idea is that if the mind manufactures the body, and if it be true that each mind is only one outlet to the infinite energy, there should be no limit to each outlet getting any amount of power from outside. Why is it impossible to keep our bodies all the time? We have to manufacture all the bodies that we ever have. As soon as this body dies, we shall have to manufacture another. If we can do that, why cannot we do it just here and now, without getting out of the present body?

The theory is perfectly correct. If it is possible that we live after death, and make other bodies, why is it impossible that we should have the power of making bodies here, without entirely dissolving this body, simply changing it continually? They also thought that in mercury and in sulphur was hidden the most wonderful power, and that by certain preparations of these a man could keep the body as long as he liked.

Others believed that certain drugs could bring powers, such as flying through the air. Many of the most wonderful medicines of the present day we owe to the Rasayana, notably the use of metal in medicine. Certain sects of yogis claim that many of their principal teachers are still living in their old bodies. Patanjali, the great authority on yoga, does not deny this.

The power of words: There are certain sacred words called Mantras, which have power, when repeated under proper conditions, to produce these extraordinary powers. We are living in the midst of such a mass of miracles, day and night, that we do not think anything of them. There is no limit to man's power, the power of words and the power of mind.

Mortification: You find that in every religion mortification and asceticism's have been practiced. In these religious conceptions the Hindus always go to extremes. You will find men with their hands up all their lives, until their hands wither and die. Men keep standing, day and night, until their feet swell, and if they live, the legs become so stiff in this position that they can no more bend them, but have to stand all their lives. I once saw a man who had kept his hands raised in this way, and I asked him how it felt when he did it first. He said it was awful torture. It was such torture that he had to go to a river and put himself in water, and that allayed the pain for a little while. After a month he did not suffer much. Through such practices powers (Siddhis) can be attained. ·

Concentration: Concentration is Samadhi, and that is yoga proper; that is the principal theme of this science, and it is the highest means. The preceding ones are only secondary, and we cannot attain to the highest through them. Samadhi is the means through which we can gain anything and everything, mental, moral or spiritual.

जात्यन्तपरिणामः प्रकृत्यापूरात् ॥2॥

The change into another species is by the filling in of nature.

Patanjali has advanced the proposition that these powers come by birth, sometimes by chemical means, or through mortification. He also admits that this body can be kept for any length of time. Now he goes on to the body into another species . He says this is done by the filling in of nature, which he explains in the next aphorism.

निमित्तप्रयोजकं प्रकृतीनां वरणभेदस्तु ततः क्षेत्रिकवत् ॥3॥

Good and bad deeds are not the direct causes in the transformations of nature, but they act as breakers of obstacles to the evolutions of nature, as a farmer breaks the obstacles to the course of water, which then runs down by its own nature.

The water for irrigation of fields is already in the canal, only shut in by gates. The farmer opens these gates, and water flows in by itself, by the law of gravitation. So all progress and power are already in every man; perfection is man's nature, only it is barred in and prevented from taking its proper course. If anyone can take the bar off, in rushes nature. Then the man attains the powers which are his already. Those we call wicked become saints, as soon as the bar is broken and nature rushes in. It is nature that is driving us towards perfection, and eventually she will bring everyone there. All these practices and struggles to become religious are only negative work, to take off the bars, and open the doors to that perfection which is our birthright, our nature.

Today the evolution theory of the ancient yogis will be better understood in the light of modern research. And yet the theory of the yogis is a better explanation. The two causes of evolution advanced by the moderns, viz. sexual selection and survival of the fittest, are inadequate. Suppose human knowledge to have advanced so much as to eliminate competition both from the function of acquiring physical sustenance and of acquiring a mate. Then, according to the moderns, human progress will stop and the race will die.

The result of this theory is to furnish every oppressor with an argument to calm the qualms of conscience. Men are not lacking, who, posing as philosophers, want to kill out all wicked and incompetent persons (they are, of course, the only judges of competency) and thus preserve the human race! But the great ancient evolutionist Patanjali, declares that the true secret of evolution is the manifestation of the perfection which is already in every being; that this perfection has been barred and the infinite tide behind is struggling to express itself.

These struggles and competitions are but the results

of our ignorance, because we do not know the proper way to unlock the gate and let the water in. This infinite tide behind must express itself; it is the cause of all manifestation. Competitions for life or sex-gratification are only momentary, unnecessary, extraneous effects, caused by ignorance. Even when all competition has ceased, this perfect nature behind will make us go forward until everyone has become perfect.

Therefore, there is no reason to believe that competition is necessary to progress. In the animal the man was suppressed, but as soon as the door was opened, out rushed man. So in man there is the potential god, kept in by the locks and bars of ignorance. When knowledge breaks these bars, the god becomes manifest.

निर्माणचित्तान्यस्मितामात्रात् ॥4॥

From egoism alone proceed the created minds.

The theory of Karma is that we suffer for our good or bad deeds, and the whole scope of philosophy is to reach the glory of man. All the scriptures sing the glory of man, of the soul, and then, in the same breath, they preach Karma. A good deed brings such a result, and a bad deed such another, but if the soul can be acted upon by a good or a bad deed, the soul amounts to nothing. Bad deeds put a bar to the manifestation of the nature of the Purusha; good deeds take the obstacles off, and the glory of the Purusha becomes manifest. The Purusha itself is never changed. Whatever you do never destroys your own glory, your own nature, because the soul cannot be acted upon by anything, only a veil is spread before it, hiding its perfection.

With a view to exhausting their Karma quickly, yogis create Kaya-vyuha, or groups of bodies, in which to work it out. For all these bodies they create minds from egoism. These are called "created minds", in contradistinction to their original minds.

प्रवृत्तिभेदे प्रयोजकं चित्तमेकमनेकेषाम् ॥5॥

Though the activities of the different created minds are various, the one original mind is the controller of them all.

These different minds, which act in these different bodies are called made-minds, and the bodies, made bodies; that is, manufactured bodies and minds. Matter and mind are like two inexhaustible storehouses. When you become a yogi, you learn the secret of their control. It was yours all the time but you had forgotten it. When you become a yogi, you recollect it. Then you can do anything with it, manipulate it in every way you like.

The material out of which a manufactured mind is created is the very same material which is used for the macrocosm. It is not that mind is one thing and matter another, they are different aspects of the same thing. Asmita, egoism is the material, the fine state of existence out of which these made-minds and made-bodies of the yogi are manufactured. Therefore, when the yogi has found the secret of these energies of nature, he can manufacture any number of bodies or minds out of the substance known as egoism.

तत्र ध्यानजमनाशयम् ॥6॥

Among the various Chittas, that which is attained by Samadhi is desireless.

Among all the various minds that we see in various men, only that mind which has attained to Samadhi, perfect concentration, is the highest. A man who has attained certain powers through medicines, or through words, or through mortifications, still has desires, but that the man who has attained to Samadhi through concentration is alone free from all desires.

कर्माशुक्लाकृष्णं योगिनस्त्रिविधमितरेषाम् ॥7॥

Works are neither black nor white for the yogis; for others they are threefold—black, white and mixed.

When the yogi has attained perfection, his actions, and the Karma produced by those actions do not bind him, because he did not desire them. He just works on; he works to do good, and he does good, but good does not care for the result, and it will not come to him. But, for ordinary men, who have not attained to that highest state, works are of three kinds, black (evil actions), white (good actions), and mixed.

ततस्तद्विपाकानुगुणानामेवाभिव्यक्तिर्वासनानाम् ॥8॥

From these threefold works are manifested in each state only those desires (which are) fitting to that state alone. (The others are held in abeyance for the time being).

Suppose I have made the three kinds of Karma, good, bad and mixed, and suppose I die and become a god in heaven. The desires in a god body are not the same as the desires in a human body; the god body neither eats nor drinks. What becomes of my past unworked Karmas which produce as their effect the desire to eat and drink? Where would these Karmas go when I become a god?

The answer is that desires can only manifest themselves in proper environments. Only those desires will come out for which the environment is fitted; the rest will remain stored up. In this life we have many godly desires, many human desires, many animal desires. If I take a god body, only the good desires will come up, because for them the environment is suitable. And if I take an animal body, only the animal desires will come up, and the good desire will wait.

What does this show? That by means of environment we can check these desires. Only that Karma which is suited to and fitted for the environment will come out. This shows that the power of environment is the great check to control even Karma itself.

जाति-देश-काल-व्यवहितानामप्यानन्तर्यं स्मृतिसंस्कारयोरेकरूपत्वात् ॥9॥

There is consecutiveness in desires, even though separated by species, space, and time, there being identification of memory and impressions.

Experiences becoming fine become impression; impressions revivified become memory. The word memory here includes unconscious coordination of past experiences, reduced to impressions, with present conscious action. In each body, the group of impressions acquired in a similar body only becomes the cause of action in that body. The experiences of a dissimilar body are held in abeyance. Each body acts as if it were a descendant of a series of bodies of that species only, thus, consecutiveness of desires is not to be broken.

तासामनादित्वं चाशिषो नित्यत्वात् ॥10॥

Thirst for happiness being eternal, desires are without beginning.

All experience is preceded by desire for happiness. There was no beginning of experience as each fresh experience is built upon the tendency generated by past experience; therefore, desire is without beginning.

हेतुफलाश्रयालम्बनैः संगृहीतत्वादेषामभावे तदभावः ॥11॥

Being held together by cause, effect, support and objects, in the absence of these is its absence.

Desires are held together by cause and effect; if a desire has been raised, it does not die without producing its effect.

Then again, the mind-stuff is the great storehouse, the support of all past desires reduced to Samskara form; until they have worked themselves out, they will not die. Moreover, so long as the sense receive the external objects, fresh desires will arise. If it be possible to get rid of the cause, effect, support, and objects of desire, then alone it will vanish.

अतीतानागतं स्वरूपतोऽस्त्यध्वभेदाद्धर्माणाम् ॥12॥

The past and future exist in their own nature, qualities having different ways.

The idea is that existence never comes out of non-existence. The past and future, though not existing in a manifested form, yet exist in a fine form.

ते व्यक्त-सूक्ष्मा गुणात्मानः ॥13॥

They are manifested or fine, being of the nature of the Gunas.

The Gunas are the three substances, Sattva, Rajas and Tamas, whose gross state is the sensible universe. Past and future arise from the different modes of manifestation of these Gunas.

परिणामैकत्वाद्वस्तुतत्वम् ॥14॥

The unity in things is from the unity in changes.

Though there are three substances, their changes being co-ordinate, all objects have their unity.

वस्तुसाम्ये चित्तभेदात्तयोर्विभक्तः पन्थाः ॥15॥

Since perception and desire vary with regard to the same object, mind and object are of different nature.

That is, there is an objective world independent of our minds. This is a refutation of Buddhistic Idealism. Since different people look at the same thing differently, it cannot be a mere imagination of any particular individual.

तदुपरागापेक्षित्वाच्चित्तस्य वस्तु ज्ञाताज्ञातम् ॥16॥

Things are known or unknown to the mind, being dependent on the colouring which they give to the mind.

सदा ज्ञाताश्चित्तवृत्तयस्तत्प्रभोः पुरुषस्यापरिणामित्वात् ॥17॥

The states of the mind are always known, because the lord of the mind, the Purusha, is unchangeable.

The whole gist of this theory is that the universe is both mental and material. Both of these are in a continuous state of flux. What is this book? One lot is going out, and another coming in; it is a whirlpool, but what makes the unity? What makes it the same book? The changes are rhythmical; in harmonious order they are sending impressions to my mind, and these pieced together make a continuous picture, although the parts are continuously changing. Mind itself is continuously changing.

The mind and body are like two layers in the same substance, moving at different rates of speed. Relatively, one being slower and the other quicker, we can distinguish between the two motion. For instance, a train is in motion, and a carriage is moving alongside it. It is possible to find the motion of both these to a certain extent. But still something else is necessary. Motion can only be perceived when there is something else which is not moving. But when two or three things are relatively moving we first perceive the motion of the faster one, and then that of the slower ones. How is the mind to perceive? It is also in a flux.

Therefore, another thing is necessary which moves more slowly, then you must get to something in which the motion is still slower, and so on, and you will find no end. Therefore, logic compels you to stop somewhere. You must complete the series by knowing something which never changes. Behind this never-ending chain of motion is the

Purusha, the impressions are merely reflected upon it, as a magic lantern throws images upon a screen, without in any way tarnishing it.

न तत् स्वाभासं दृश्यत्वात् ॥18॥

The mind is not self-luminous, being an object.

Tremendous power is manifested everywhere in nature, but it is not self-luminous, not essentially intelligent. The Purusha alone is self-luminous, and gives its light to everything. It is the power of the Purusha that is percolating through all matter and force.

एकसमये चोभयानवधारणम् ॥19॥

From its being unable to cognise both at the same time.

If the mind were self-luminous it would be able to cognise itself and its objects at the same time, which it cannot. When it cognises the objects, it cannot reflect on itself. Therefore, the Purusha is self-luminous, and the mind is not.

चित्तान्तरदृश्ये बुद्धिबुद्धेरतिप्रसङ्गः स्मृतिसङ्करश्च ॥20॥

Another cognising mind being assumed, there will be no end to such assumptions, and confusion of memory will be the result.

Let us suppose there is another mind which cognises the ordinary mind, then there will have to be still another to cognise the former, and so there will be no end to it. It will result in confusion of memory, there will be no storehouse of memory.

चितेरप्रतिसक्रमायास्तदाकारपत्तौ स्वबुद्धिसंवेदनम् ॥21॥

The essence of knowledge (the Purusha) being unchangeable, when the mind takes its form, it becomes conscious.

Patanjali says this to make it more clear that knowledge is not a quality of the Purusha. When the mind comes near the Purusha it is reflected, as it were upon the mind, and the mind, for the time being becomes knowing and seems as if it were itself the Purusha.

द्रष्टृदृश्योपरक्तं चित्तं सर्वार्थम् ॥22॥

Coloured by the seer and the seen the mind is able to understand everything.

On one side of the mind the external world, the seen is being reflected, and on the other, the seer is being reflected. Thus comes the power of all knowledge to the mind.

तदसंख्येयवासनाभिश्चित्रमपि परार्थं संहत्यकारित्वात् ॥23॥

The mind, though variegated by innumerable desires, acts for another (the Purusha), because it acts in combination.

The mind is a compound of various things and therefore it cannot work for itself. Everything that is a combination in this world has some objects for that combination, some third thing for which this combination is going on. So this combination of the mind is for the Purusha.

विशेषदर्शिन आत्मभाव-भावनानिवृत्तिः ॥24॥

For the discriminating, the perception of the mind as Atman ceases.

Through discrimination the yogi knows that the Purusha is not mind.

तदा विवेकनिम्नं कैवल्यप्रागभाव चित्तम् ॥25॥

Then, bent on discriminating the mind attains the previous state of Kaivalya (isolation).

Thus the practice of yoga leads to discriminating power,

to clearness of vision. The veil drops from the eyes, and we see things as they are. We find that nature is a compound, and is showing the panorama for the Purusha, who is the witness. That nature is not the Lord, that all the combination of nature are simply for the sake of showing these phenomena to the Purusha, the enthroned king within. When discrimination comes by long practice, fear ceases, and the mind attains isolation.

तच्छिद्रेषु प्रत्ययान्तराणि संस्कारेभ्यः ॥26॥

The thoughts that arise as obstructions to that are from impressions.

All the various ideas that arise, making us believe that we require something external to make us happy, are obstructions to that perfection. The Purusha is happiness and blessedness by its own nature. But that knowledge is covered over by past impressions. These impressions have to work themselves out.

हानमेषां क्लेशवदुक्तम् ॥27॥

Their destruction is in the same manner as of ignorance, egoism, etc., as said before (II.10).

प्रसंख्यानेऽप्यकुसीदस्य सर्वथा विवेकख्यातेर्धर्ममेघः समाधिः ॥28॥

Even when arriving at the right discriminating knowledge of the essences, he who gives up the fruits, unto him comes, as the result of perfect discrimination, the Samadhi called the cloud of virtue.

When the yogi has attained to this discrimination, all the powers mentioned in the last chapter come to him, but the true yogi rejects them all. Unto him comes a peculiar knowledge, a particular light, called the Dharmamegha, the cloud of virtue. All the great prophets of the world whom history has recorded had this. They had found the whole foundation of knowledge within themselves. Truth to them had become real. Peace and calmness, and perfect purity became their own nature, after they had given up the vanities of powers.

ततः क्लेशकर्मनिवृत्तिः ॥29॥

From that comes cessation of pain and works.

When the cloud of virtue has come, then no more is there fear of falling, nothing can drag the yogi down. No more will there be evils for him. No more pains.

तदा सर्वावरणमलापेतस्य ज्ञानस्याऽनन्त्याज्ज्ञेयमल्पम् ॥30॥

Then knowledge, bereft of covering and impurities, becoming infinite, the knowable becomes small.

Knowledge itself is there; its covering is gone. One of the Buddhist scriptures defines what is meant by the Buddha (which is the name of a state) as infinite knowledge, infinite as the sky. Jesus attained to that and became the Christ. All of you will attain to that state. Knowledge becoming infinite, the knowable becomes small. The whole universe, with all its objects of knowledge, becomes as nothing before the Purusha. The ordinary man thinks himself very small, because to him knowable seems to be infinite.

ततः कृतार्थानां परिणामक्रमसमाप्तिर्गुणानाम् ॥31॥

Then are finished the successive transfor-mations of the qualities, they having attained the end.

Then all these various transformations of the qualities, which change from species to species, cease for ever.

क्षणप्रतियोगी परिणामापरान्तनिर्ग्राह्यः क्रमः ॥32॥

The changes that exist in relation to moments and which are perceived at the other end (at the end of a series) are succession.

Patanjali here defines the word succession, the changes that exist in relation to moments. While I think, many moments pass, and with each moment there is a change of idea, but I only perceive these changes at the end of a series. This is called succession, but for the mind that has realised omnipresence there is no succession. Everything has become present for it; to it the present alone exists, the past and future are lost. Time stands controlled, all knowledge is there in one second. Everything is known like a flash.

पुरुषार्थशून्यानां गुणानां प्रतिप्रसवः कैवल्यं स्वरूपप्रतिष्ठा वा चितिशक्तेरिति ॥33॥

The resolution in the inverse order of the qualities, bereft of any motive of action for the Purusha, is Kaivalya, or it is the establishment of the power of knowledge in its own nature.

Nature's task is done, this unselfish task which our sweet nurse, nature, had imposed upon herself. She gently took the self-forgetting soul by the hand, as it were, and showed him all the experiences in the universe, all manifestations, bringing him higher and higher through various bodies, till his lost glory came back, and he remembered his own nature. Then the kind mother went back the same way she came, for others who also have lost their way in the trackless desert of life. And thus is she working, without beginning and without end. And thus through pleasure and pain, through good and evil, the infinite river of souls is flowing into the ocean of perfection, of self-realisation.

Glory unto those who have realised their own nature. May their blessings be on us all!

III

Simple Lessons in RAJAYOGA

Six Lessons for Practice

These lessons were given by Swami Vivekananda to some of his devoted American students at the residence of his disciple Mrs. Sara C. Bull some time in the last decade of the 19th century. These were preserved by her, and two decades later, published by her for the benefit of those who would be interested. Its Indian edition was published in 1928 by Udbodhan Office, Calcutta.

This happens to be the most useful course for learners, especially in present times when yoga has become a rage in most enlightened countries.

To the Student

Rajayoga is as much a science as any in the world. It is an analysis of the mind, gathering the facts of the super-sensuous world and so building up the spiritual world. All the great spiritual teachers the world has known, said, 'I see and I know. Jesus, Paul and Peter all claimed actual perception of the spiritual truths they taught.

This perception is obtained be yoga.

Neither memory nor consciousness can be the limitation of existence. There is a superconscious state. Both it and the unconscious state are sensationless, but with a vast difference between them—the difference between ignorance and knowledge. Present yoga is an appeal to reason, as a science.

Concentration of the mind is the source of all knowledge.

Yoga teaches us to make matter our slave, as it ought to be. Yoga means 'yoke', 'to join', that is, to join the soul of man with the supreme Soul of God.

Mind acts in and under consciousness. What we call consciousness is only one link in the infinite chain that is our nature.

This 'I' of ours covers just a little consciousness and a vast amount of unconsciousness, while over it, and mostly unknown to it, is the superconscious plane.

Through faithful practice, layer after layer of mind opens before us, and each reveals new facts to us. We see as it were new worlds created before us, new powers are put into our hands, but we must not stop by the way, or allow ourselves to be dazzled by these 'beads of glass' when the mine of diamonds lies before us.

God alone is our goal. Failing to reach God, we die.

Three things are necessary to the student who wishes to succeed.

First, give up all ideas of enjoyment in this world and the next, care only for God and Truth. We are here to know truth, not for enjoyment. Leave that to brutes who enjoy as we never can. Man is a thinking being and must struggle on until he conquers death, until he sees the light. He must not spend himself in vain talking that bears no fruit. Worship of society and popular opinion is idolatry. The soul has no sex, no country, no place, no time.

Second, intense desire to know Truth and God. Be eager for them, long for them, as a drawing man longs for breath. Want only God, take nothing else, let not 'seeming' cheat you any longer. Turn from all and seek only God.

Third, the first—Restraining the mind from going outward. Second—Restraining the sense. Third—Turning the mind inward. Fourth—Suffering everything without murmuring. Fifth— Fastening the mind to one idea. Take the subject before you and think it out; never leave it. Do not count time. Sixth—Think constantly of your real nature. Get rid of superstition. Do not hypnotize yourself into a belief in your own inferiority. Day and night tell yourself what you really are, until you realize (actually realise) your oneness with God. Without these disciplines, no results can be gained.

We can be conscious of the Absolute, but we can never express it. The moment we try to express It, we limit it and it ceases to be absolute. We have to go beyond sense limit and transcend even reason, and we have the power to do this.

First Lesson

This is a lesson seeking to bring out the individuality. Each individuality must be cultivated. All will meet at the centre. Imagination is the door to inspiration and the basis of all thought.' All prophets, poets and discoverers have had great imaginative power. The explanation of nature is in us; the stone falls outside, but gravitation is in us, not outside. Those who stuff themselves, those who starve themselves, those who sleep too much, those who sleep too little, cannot become yogis. Ignorance, fickleness, jealousy, laziness, and excessive attachment are the great enemies to success in yoga practice. The three great requisites are:

First, purity: physical and mental; all uncleanness, all that would draw the mind down, must be abandoned.

Second, patience: At first there will be wonderful manifestations, but they will all cease. This is the hardest period, but hold fast; in the end the gain is sure if you have patience.

Third, perseverance: Persevere through thick and thin, through health and sickness, never miss a day in practice.

The best time for practice is the junction of day and night, the calmest time in the tides of our bodies, the zero point between two states. If this cannot be done, practise upon rising and going to bed. Great personal cleanliness is necessary—a daily bath.

After bathing, sit down and hold the seat firm., that is, imagine that you sit as firm as a rock, that nothing can move you. Hold the head and shoulders and the hips in straight line, keeping the spinal column free: all action is along it, and must not be impaired.

Begin with your toes and think of each part of your body as perfect; picture it so in your mind, touching each part if you prefer to do so. Pass upward, bit by bit, until you reach the head, thinking of each as perfect, lacking nothing. Then think of the whole as perfect, an instrument given to you by God to enable you to attain Truth. The vessel in which you are to cross the ocean and reach the shores of eternal truth. When this has been done, take a long breath through both nostrils, throw it out again, and then hold it out as long as you comfortably can. Take four such breaths, then breathe naturally and pray for illumination.

'I meditate on the glory of that being who created this universe; may he illuminate my mind'. Sit and meditate on this ten or fifteen minutes.

Tell your experiences to no one but your Guru.

Talk as little as possible.

Keep your thoughts on virtue; what we think we tend to become.

Holy meditation helps to burn out all mental impurities. All who are not yogis are slaves; bond after bond must be broken to make us free.

All can find the reality beyond. If God is true, we must feel him as a fact, and if there is a soul, we ought to be able to see it and feel it.

The only way to find if there be a soul is to be something which is not the body.

The yogis class our organs under two chief heads: organs of sense and organs of motion, or knowledge and action.

The internal organ or mind has four aspects. First—Manas, the cogitating or thinking faculty, which is usually almost entirely wasted, because uncontrolled; properly governed, it is a wonderful power. Second—Buddhi, the will (sometimes called the intellect). Third—Ahamkara, the self-conscious egotism (from Aham). Fourth—Chitta, the substance in and through which all the faculties act, the floor of the mind as it were, or the sea in which the various faculties are waves.

Yoga is the science by which we stop Chitta from assuming, or becoming transformed into several faculties. As the reflection of the moon on the sea is broken or blurred by the waves, so is the reflection of the Atman, the true Self, broken by the mental waves. Only when the sea is stilled to mirror-like calmness can the reflection of the moon be seen, and only when the 'mind-stuff', the Chitta, is controlled to absolute calmness is the Self to be recognized.

The mind is not the body, though it is matter in a finer form. It is not eternally bound by the body. This is proved as we get occasionally loosened from it. We can learn to do this at will by controlling the senses.

When we can do that fully, we shall control the universe, because our world is only what the senses bring us. Freedom is the test of the higher being. Spiritual life begins when you have loosened yourself from the control of the senses. He whose senses rule him is worldly—is a slave.

If we could entirely stop our mind-stuff from breaking into waves, it would put an end to our bodies. For millions of years we have worked so hard to manufacture these bodies that in the struggle we have forgotten our real purpose in getting them, which was to become perfect. We have grown to think that body-making is the end of our efforts. This is Maya. We must break this delusion and return to our original aim and realize we are not the body, it is our servant.

Learn to take the mind out and to see that it is separate from the body. We endow the body with sensation and life and then think it is alive and real. We have worn it so long that we forget that it is not identical with us. Yoga is to help us put off our body when we please and see it as our servant, out instrument, not our ruler. Controlling the mental powers is the first great aim in yoga practices. The second is concentrating them in full force upon any subject.

You cannot be a yogi if you talk much.

Second Lesson

This yoga is known as the eightfold yoga, because it is divided into eight principal parts. These are:

First—Yama. This is most important and has to govern the whole life; it has five divisions:

1st. Not injuring any being by thought, word, or deed.
2nd. Non-covetousness in thought, word, or deed.
3rd. Perfect chastity in thought, word, or deed.
4th. Perfect truthfulness in thought, word, or deed.
5th. Non-receiving of gifts.

Second—Niyama. The bodily care, bathing daily, dietary, etc.

Third—Asana. Posture. Hips, shoulders, and head must be held straight, leaving the spine free.

Fourth—Pranayama. Restraining the breath (in order to get control of the Prana or vital force).

Fifth—Pratyahara. Turning the mind inward and restraining it from going outward, revolving the matter in the mind in order to understand it.

Sixth—Dharana. Concentration on one subject.

Seventh—Dhyana. Meditation.

Eight—Samadhi. Illumination, the aim of all our efforts.

Yama and Niyama are for lifelong practice; as for the others, we do as the leech does, not leave one blade of grass before firmly grasping another. In other words, we have thoroughly to understand and practise one step before taking another.

The subject of this lesson is Pranayama, or controlling

Prana. In Rajayoga breathing enters the psychic plane and brings us to the spiritual. It is the fly-wheel of the whole bodily system. It acts first upon the lungs, the lungs act on the heart, the heart acts upon the circulation, this in turn upon the brain, and the brain upon the mind. The will can produce and arouse the will. Our wills are weak; we do not realize their power, we are so much bound up in matter. Most of our action is from outside in. Outside nature throws us off our balance and we cannot (as we ought) throw nature off her balance. This is all wrong; the stronger power is really within.

The great saints and teachers were those who had conquered this world of thought within thcmselves and so spake with power. The story of the minister confined in a high tower, who was brought him a beetle, honey, a silken thread, a cord, and a rope, illustrates the way we gain control of our mind by using first the physical regulation of the breath as the silken thread. That enables us to lay hold of one power after another until the rope of concentration delivers us from the prison of the body and we are free. Reaching freedom, we can discard the means used to bring us there.

Pranayama has three parts:

1st. Puraka—inhaling.

2nd.Kumbhaka—restraining.

3rd. Rechaka—exhaling.

There are two currents passing through the brain and circulating down the sides of the spine, crossing at the base and returing to the brain. One of these currents, called the 'Sun' (Pingala), starts from the left hemisphere of the brain, crosses at the base of the brain to the right side of the spine, and recrosses at the base of the spine, like one-half of the figure eight.

The other current, the 'moon' (Ida), reverses this action

and completes the figure eight. Of course, the lower part is much longer than the upper. These currents flow day and night and make deposits of the great life forces at different points, commonly known as 'plexuses'; but we are rarely conscious of them. By concentration we can learn to feel them and trace them over all parts of the body. These 'sun' and "moon' currents are intimately connected with breathing, and by regulating this we get control of the body.

In the *Katha Upanishad* the body is described as the chariot, the mind is the reins, the intellect is the charioteer, the senses are the horses, and the objects of the senses their road. The self is the rider, seated in the chariot. Unless the rider has understanding and can make the charioteer control his horses, he can never attain the goal; but the senses, like vicious steeds, will drag him where they please and may even destroy him. These two currents are the great 'check rein' in the hands of the charioteer, and he must get control of this to control the horses. We have to get the power to become moral; until we do that, we cannot control our actions. Yoga alone enables us to carry into practice the teachings of morality. To become moral is the object of yoga. All great teachers were yogis and controlled every current. The yogis arrest these currents at the base of the spine and force them through the centre of the spinal column. They then become the current of knowledge, which only exists in the yogi.

Second Lesson in breathing: One method is not for all. This breathing must be done with rhythmic regularity, and the easiest way is by counting; as that is purely mechanical, we repeat the sacred word 'Om' a certain number of times instead.

The process of Pranayama is as follows: Close the right nostril with thumb and then slowly inhale through the left nostril, repeating the word 'Om' eight times.

Then, removing the thumb from the right nostril, exhale slowly through that, repeating 'Om' four times.

As you close the exhalation, draw in the abdomen forcibly to expel all the air from the lungs. Then slowly inhale through the right nostril, keeping the left one closed, repeating 'Om' four times. Next close the right nostril with the thumb and hold the breath while repeating 'Om' eight times. Then unclose the left nostril and slowly exhale, repeating 'Om' four times, drawing in the abdomen as before. Repeat this whole operation twice at each sitting, that is, making four Pranayamas, two for each nostril. Before taking your seat it is well to begin with prayer.

This needs to be practised a week; then gradually increase the duration of breathings, keeping the same ratio, that is, if you repeat 'Om' six times at inhalation, then do the same at exhalation and twelve times during Kumbhaka. These exercises will make us more spiritual, more pure, more holy. Do not be led aside into any byways or seek after power. Love is the only power that stays by us and increases. He who seeks to come to God through Rajayoga must be strong mentally, physical, morally, and spiritually. Take every step in that light.

Third Lesson

Kundalini : Realize the soul not as matter, but as it is. We are thinking of the soul as body, but we must separate it from sense and thought. Then alone can we know we are immortal. Change implies the duality of cause and effect, and all that changes must be mortal. This proves that the body cannot be immortal, nor can the mind, because both are constantly changing. Only the unchangeable can be immortal, because there is nothing to act upon it.

We do not become it, we are it; but we have to clear away the veil of ignorance that hides the truth from us. The body is objectified thought. The 'sun' and 'moon' currents bring energy to all parts of the body. The surplus energy is stored at certain points (plexuses) along the spinal column commonly known as nerve centers.

These currents are not to be found in dead bodies and can only be traced in a healthy organism.

The yogi has an advantage; for he is able not only to feel them, but actually to see them. They are luminous in his life, and so are the great nerve centres.

There is conscious as well as unconscious action. The yogis posses a third kind, the super conscious, which in all countries and in all ages has been the source of all religious knowledge. The superconscious state makes no mistakes, but whereas the action of the instinct would be purely mechanical, the former is beyond consciousness. It has been called inspiration, but the yogi says, 'This faculty is in every human being, and eventually all will enjoy it'.

We must give a new direction to the 'sun' and 'moon'

currents and open for them a new passage through the centre of the spinal cord. When we succeed in bringing the currents through this passage called Sushumna, up to the brain, we are for the time being separated entirely from the body.

The nerve centre at the base of the spine near the sacrum is most important. It is the seat of the generative substance of the sexual energy and is symbolised by the yogi as a triangle containing a tiny serpent coiled up in it. The sleeping serpent is called Kundalini and to raise the Kundalini is the whole object or Rajayoga.

The great sexual force, raised from animal action and sent upward to the great dynamo of the human system, the brain, and there stored up, becomes Ojas or spiritual force. All good thought, all prayer, resolves a part of that animal energy into Ojas and helps to give us spiritual power. This Ojas is the real man and in human beings alone is it possible for this storage of Ojas to be accomplished. One in whom the whole animal sex force has been transformed into Ojas is a God. He speaks with power, and his words regenerate the world.

The yogi pictures this serpent as being slowly lifted from stage to stage until the highest, the pineal gland, is reached. No man or woman can be really spiritual until the sexual energy, the highest power possessed by man, has been converted into Ojas.

No force can be created; it can only be directed. Therefore, we must learn to control the grand powers that are already in our hands and by will power make them spiritual instead of merely animal. Thus it is clearly seen that chastity is the cornerstone of all morality and of all religion. In Raja-yoga especially, absolute chastity in thought, word, and deed is a *sine qua non.* The same laws apply to the married and the single. If one wastes the most potent forces of one's being cannot become spiritual.

All history teaches us that the great seers of all ages were either monks and ascetics or those who had given up married life; only the pure in life can see God.

Just before making the Pranayama, endeavour to visualise the triangle. Close your eyes and picture it vividly in your imagination. See it surrounded by flames and with the serpent coiled in the middle. When you can clearly see the Kundalini; place it in imagination at the base of the spine, and when restraining the breath in Kumbhaka, throw it forcibly down on the head of the serpent to awaken it. The more powerful the imagination, the more quickly will the real result be attained and the Kundalini be awakened. Until it does, imagine it does: try to feel the currents and try to force them through the Sushumna. This hastens their action.

Fourth Lesson

Before we can control the mind we must study it. We have to seize this unstable mind and drag it from its wanderings and fix it on one idea. Over and over again this must be done. By power of will we must get hold of the mind and make it stop and reflect upon the glory of God.

The easiest way to get hold of the mind is to sit quiet and let it drift where is will for a while. Hold fast to the idea, 'I am the witness watching my mind drifting. The mind is not I.' Then see it think as if it were a thing entirely apart from yourself. Identify yourself with God, never with matter or with the mind.

Picture the mind as a calm lake stretched before you and the thoughts that come and go as bubbles rising and breaking on its surface. Make no effort to control them in imagination as they float away. This will gradually lessen the circles. For the mind ranges over wide circles of thought and those circles widen out into ever-increasing circles, as in a pond when we throw a stone into it. We want to reverse the process and starting with a huge circle make it narrower until at last we can fix the mind on one point and make it stay there. Hold to the idea, 'I am not the mind, I see that I am thinking, I am watching my mind act', and each day the identification of yourself with thought and feeling will grow less, until at last you can entirely separate yourself from the mind and actually know it to be apart from yourself.

When this is done, the mind is your servant to control as you will. The first stage of being a yogi is to go beyond the senses. When the mind is conquered, he has reached the highest stage. Live alone as much as possible. The seat should be of comfortable height; pur first a grass mat, then a skin (fur), next a silken cover. It is better that the seat has no back and it must stand firm.

Thoughts being pictures, we should not create them. We have to exclude all thought from the mind and make it a blank; as fast as a thought comes we have to banish it. To be able to accomplish this, we must transcend matter and go beyond our body. The whole life of man is really an effort to do this.

Each sound has its own meaning. In our nature these two things are connected.

The highest ideal we have is God. Meditate on Him. We cannot know the Knower, but we are He.

Seeing evil, we are creating it. What we are we see outside, for the world is our mirror. This little body is a little mirror we have created, but the whole universe is our body. We must think this all the time; then we shall know that we cannot die or hurt another, because he is our own. We are birthless and deathless and we ought only to love.

'This whole universe is my body; all health, all happiness is mine, because all is in the universe.' Say, 'I am the universe.' We finally learn that all action is from us to the mirror.

Although we appear as little waves, the whole sea is at our back and we are one with it. No wave can exist of itself.

Imagination properly employed is our greatest friend; it goes beyond reason and is the only light that takes us everywhere.

Inspiration is from within and we have to inspire ourselves by our own higher faculties.

Fifth Lesson

Pratyahara and Dharana: Krishna says, 'All who seek me by whatever means will reach me.' 'All must reach me.' Pratyahara is gathering toward, an attempt to get hold of the mind and focus it on the desired object. The first step is to let the mind drift; watch it; see what it thinks: be only the witness. Mind is not soul or spirit. It is only matter in a finer form, and we own it and can learn to manipulate it through the nerve energies.

The body is the objective view of what we call mind (subjective). We, the Self, are beyond both body and mind; we are Atman, the eternal unchangeable witness. The body is crystallised thought.

When the breath is flowing through the left nostril, it is the time for rest; when through the right, for work; and when through both, the time to meditate. When we are calm and breathing equally through both nostrils, we are in the right condition for quiet meditation. It is no use trying to concentrate at first. Control of thought will come of itself.

After sufficient practice of closing the nostrils with the thumb and forefinger, we shall be able to do it by the power of will, through thought alone.

Pranayama is now to be slightly changed. If the student has the name of his Ishta (Chosen Ideal) he should use that instead of Om during inhalation and exhalation, and use the word Hum (pronounced Hooe) during Kumbhaka.

Throw the restrained breath forcibly down on the head of the Kundalini at each repetition of the word Hum and imagine that this awakens her. Identify yourself only with

God. After a while thoughts will announce their coming, and we shall learn the way they begin and be aware of what we are going to think, just as on this plane we can look out and see a person coming. This stage is reached when we have learnt to separate ourselves from our minds and see ourselves as one and thought as something apart. Do not let the thoughts grasp you; stand aside and they will die away.

Follow these holy thoughts; go with them; and when they melt away you will find the feet of the Omnipotent God. This is the superconscious state; when out the idea melts, follow it and melt with it.

Haloes are symbols of inner light and can be seen by the yogi. Sometimes we may see a face as if surrounded by flames and in them read the character and judge without erring. We may have our Ishta come to us as a vision, and this symbol will be the one upon which we can rest easily and fully concentrate our minds.

We can imagine through all the senses, but we do so mostly through the eyes. Even imagination is half material. In other words, it is probable that there is no inseparable connection between thought and images.

Try to keep up the imagination in yoga, being careful to keep it pure and holy. We all have our peculiarities in the way of imaginative power; follow the way most natural to you; it will be easiest.

We are the result of all reincarnations through Karma; 'One lamp lighted from another;' says the Buddhist—different lamps, but the same light.

Be cheerful, be brave, bathe daily, having patience, purity and preference, then you will become a yogi in truth. Never try to hurry, and, if the higher powers come, remember that they are but side-paths. Do not let them tempt you from the main road; put them aside and hold fast to your only true aim—God. Seek only the Eternal, finding which we are at rest for ever; having the all, nothing is left to strive for, and we are for ever in free and perfect existence—Existence absolute, Knowledge absolute, Bliss absolute.

Sixth Lesson

Sushumna: It is very useful to meditate on the Sushumna. You may have a vision of it come to you and this is the best way. Then meditate for a long time on that. It is a very fine, very brilliant thread, this living passage through the spinal cord, this way of salvation through which we have to make the Kundalini rise.

In the language of the yogi, the Sushumna has its ends in two lotuses, the lower lotus surrounding the triangle of the Kundalini and the top one in the brain surrounding the pineal gland; between these two are four other lotuses, stages on the way:

6th. Pineal gland.
5th. Between the eyes.
4th. Bottom of the throat.
3rd. Level with the heart.
2nd. Opposite the navel.
1st. Base of spine.

We must awaken the Kundalini, and then slowly raise it from one lotus to another till the brain is reached. Each stage corresponds to a new layer of the mind.

IV

RAJAYOGA in Other Scriptures

In Shvetashvatara Upanishad

अग्निर्यत्राभिमथ्यते वायुर्यत्राधिरुध्यते ।
सोमो यत्रातिरिच्यते तत्र सञ्जायते मनः॥

Where the fire is rubbed, where the air is controlled, where the Soma flows over, there a (perfect) mind is created.

त्रिरुन्नतं स्थाप्य समं शरीरं हृदीन्द्रियाणि मनसा सन्निवेश्य ।
ब्रह्मोडुपेन प्रतरेत विद्वान् स्रोतांसि सर्वाणि भयावहानि ॥

Placing the body in a straight posture, with the chest, the throat, and the head held erect. Making the organs enter the mind, the sage crosses all the fearful currents by means of the raft of Brahman.

प्राणान् प्रपीड्येह संयुक्तचेष्टः क्षीणे प्राणे नासिकयोच्छ्वसीत ।
दुष्टाश्वयुक्तमिव वाहमेनं विद्वान् मनो धारयेताप्रमत्तः ॥

The man of well-regulated endeavours controls the Prana; and when it has become quieted, breathes out through the nostrils. The persevering sage holds his mind as a charioteer holds the restive horses.

समे शुचौ शर्करावह्निवालुकाविवर्जिते शब्दजलाश्रयादिभिः ।
मनोनुकूले न च चक्षुपीडने गुहानिवाताश्रयणे प्रयोजयेत् ॥

In (lonely) places as mountain caves where the floor is even, free of pebbles, fire, or sand, where there are no disturbing noises from men or waterfalls, in auspicious places helpful to the mind and pleasing to the eyes, yoga is to be practised (mind is to be joined).

नीहारधूमार्कानिलानलानां खद्योतविद्युत्-स्फटिक-शशीनाम्।
एतानि रूपाणि पुरःसराणि ब्रह्मण्यभिव्यक्तिकराणि योगे॥

Like snowfall, smoke, sun, wind, fire, firefly, lightning, crystal, moon, these forms, coming before, gradually manifest the Brahman in yoga.

पृथ्व्यप्तेजोऽनिलखे समुत्थिते पञ्चात्मके योगगुणे प्रवृत्ते।
न तस्य रोगो न जरा न मृत्युः प्राप्तस्य योगाग्निमयं शरीरम्॥

When the perceptions of yoga, arising from earth, water, light, fire, ether, have taken place, then yoga has begun. Unto him does not come disease, nor old age, nor death, who has got a body made up of the fire of yoga.

लघुत्वमारोग्यमलोलुपत्वं वर्णप्रसादः स्वरसौष्ठवञ्च।
गन्धः शुभो मूत्रपुरीषमल्पं योगप्रवृत्तिं प्रथमां वदन्ति॥

The first signs of entering yoga are lightness, health, non-covetousness, clearness of complexion, a beautiful voice, an agreeable odour in the body, and scantiness of excretions. As gold or silver, first covered with earth, and then cleaned, shines full of light, so the embodied man seeing the truth of the Atman as one, attains the goal and becomes sorrowless.

(Ch.2)

आसनानि समभ्यस्य वाञ्छितानि यथाविधि।
प्राणायामं ततो गार्गि जितासनगतोऽभ्यसेत्॥

मृद्वासने कुशान् सम्यगास्तीर्याजिनमेव च।
लम्बोदरं च सम्पूज्य फलमोदकभक्षणैः॥
तदासने सुखासीनः सव्ये न्यस्येतरं करम्।
समग्रीव शिराः सम्यक् संवृतास्यः सुनिश्चलः॥
प्राङ्मुखोदङ्मुखो वाऽपि नासाग्रन्यस्तलोचनः।
अतिभुक्तमभुक्तं वा वर्जयित्वा प्रयत्नतः॥
नाडीसंशोधनं कुर्यादुक्तमार्गेण यत्नतः।
वृथा क्लेशो भवेत्तस्य तच्छोधनमकुर्वतः॥
नासाग्रे शशभृद्बीजं चन्द्रातपवितानितम्।
सप्तमस्य तु वर्गस्य चतुर्थं बिन्दुसंयुतम्॥
विश्वमध्यस्थमालोक्य नासाग्रे चक्षुषी उभे।
इडया पूरयेद्वायुं बाह्यं द्वादशमात्रकैः॥
ततोऽग्निं पूर्ववद्ध्यायेत् स्फुरज्ज्वालावलीयुतम्।
रुषष्ठं बिन्दुसंयुक्तं शिखिमण्डलसंस्थितम्॥
ध्यायेद्विरेचयेद्वायुं मन्दं पिङ्गलया पुनः।
पुनः पिङ्गलयापूर्य घ्राणं दक्षिणतः सुधीः॥
तद्वद्विरेचयेद्वायुमिडया तु शनैः शनैः।
त्रिचतुर्वत्सरं चापि त्रिचतुर्मासमेव वा॥
गुरुणोक्तप्रकारेण रहस्येवं समभ्यसेत्।
प्रातर्मध्यन्दिने सायं स्नात्वा षट्कृत्व आचरेत्॥
सन्ध्यादिकर्म कृत्वैव मध्यरात्रेऽपि नित्यशः।
नाड़ीशुद्धिमवाप्नोति तच्चिह्नं दृश्यते पृथक्॥
शरीरलघुता दीप्तिर्जठराग्निविवर्धनम्।
नादाभिव्यक्तिरित्येतल्लिङ्गं तच्छुद्धिसूचनम्॥
प्राणायामं ततः कुर्याद्रेचकपूरककुम्भकैः।
प्राणापानसमायोगः प्राणायामः प्रकीर्तितः॥

पूरयेत् षोडशैमत्रैरापादतलमस्तकम् ।
मात्रैर्द्वात्रिंशकैः पश्चाद्रेचयेत् सुसमाहितः ॥
सम्पूर्णकुम्भवद्वायुर्निश्चलं मूर्ध्नि देशतः ।
कुम्भकं धारणं गार्गि चतुःषष्ट्या तु मात्रया ॥
ऋषयस्तु वदन्त्यन्ये प्राणायामपरायणाः ।
पवित्रीभूताः पूतान्त्राः प्रभञ्जनजये रताः ॥
तत्रादौ कुम्भकं कृत्वा चतुःषष्ट्या तु मात्रया ।
रेचयेत् षोडशैर्मात्रैर्नासेनैकेन सुन्दरि ।
ततश्च पूरयेद्वायुं शनैः षोडशमात्रया ॥
प्राणायामैर्दहेद्दोषान् धारणाभिश्च किल्बिषान् ।
प्रत्याहाराच्च संसर्गान्ध्यानेनानीश्वरान् गुणान् ॥

After practising the postures as desired, according to rules, then, O Gargi, the man who has conquered the posture will practise Pranayama.

Seated in an easy posture, on a (deer or tiger) skin, placed on Kusha grass, worshipping Ganapati with fruits and sweetmeats, placing the right palm on the left, holding the throat and head in the same line, the lips closed and firm, facing the east or the north, the eyes fixed on the tip of the nose, avoiding too much food of fasting, the Nadis should be purified without which the practice will be fruitless. Thinking of the (seedword) 'Hum', at the junction of Pingala and Ida (the right and the left nostrils), the Ida should be filled with external air in twelve Matras (seconds); then the yogi meditates on fire in the same place with the word 'Rung', and while meditating thus, slowly ejects the air through the Pingala (right nostril). Again filling in through the Pingala the air should be slowly ejected through the Ida, in the same way. This should be practised for three or four years, or three or four months, according to the directions of a Guru, in secret (alone in a room), in the early morning, at midday, in the evening, and at midnight (until) the nerves become purified. Lightness of body, clear complexion, good appetite, hearing of the Nada, are the signs of the purification of nerves. Then should be practised Pranayama composed of Rechaka (exhalation), Kumbhaka (retention), and Puraka (inhalation). Joining the Prana with the Apana is Pranayama.

In sixteen Matras filling the body from the head to the feet, in thirty-two Matras the Prana is to be thrown out, and with sixty-four the Kumbhaka should be made.

There is another Pranayama in which the Kumbhaka should first be made with sixty-four Matras, then the Prana should be thrown out with sixteen, and the body next filled with sixteen Matras.

By Pranayama impurities of the body are thrown out; by Dharana the impurities of the mind; by Pratyahara the impurities of attachment; and by Samadhi is taken off everything that hides the lordship of the Soul.

In Sankhya Karika

भावनोपचयात् शुद्धस्य सर्वं प्रकृतिवत् ॥

By the achievement of meditation, there come to the pure one (the Purusha) all powers of nature.

रागोपहतिर्ध्यानम् ॥

Meditation is the removal of attachment.

वृत्तिनिरोधात्तत्सिद्धिः ॥

It is perfected by the suppression of the modifications.

धारणाऽऽसनस्वकर्मणा तत्सिद्धिः ॥

By Dharana, posture, and performance of one's duties, it is perfected.

निरोधश्छर्दिविधारणाभ्याम् ॥

Restraint of the Prana is by means of expulsion and retention.

स्थिरसुखमासनम् ॥

Posture is that which is steady and easy.

वैराग्यादभ्यासाच्च ॥

Also by non-attachment and practice meditation is perfected.

तत्त्वाभ्यासान्नेति नेतीति त्यागाद्विवेकसिद्धिः ॥

By reflection on the principles of nature, and by

giving them up as "not It, not It", discrimi-nation is perfected.

(Book 3)

आवृत्तिरसकृदुपदेशात् ॥

Instruction is to be repeated.

श्येनवत् सुखदुःखी त्यागवियोगाभ्याम् ॥

As the hawk becomes unhappy if the food is taken away from him and happy if he gives it up himself (so he gives up everything voluntarily is happy).

अहिनिर्ल्वयनीवत् ॥

As the snake is happy in giving up his old skin.

असाधनानुचिन्तनं बन्धाय भरतवत् ॥

That which is not a means of liberation is not to be thought of; it becomes a cause of bondage, as in the case of Bharata.

बहुभिर्योगे विरोधो रागादिभिः कुमारीशङ्खवत् ॥

From the association of many things there is obstruction to meditation, through passion, aversion, etc., like the shell bracelets on the virgin's hand.

द्वाभ्यामपि तथैव ॥

It is the same even in the case of two.

निराशःसुखी पिङ्गलावत् ॥

The renouncers of hope are happy, like the girl Pingala.

बहुशास्त्रगुरूपासनेऽपि सारादानं षट्पदवत् ॥

Although devotion is to be given to many institutes and teachers, the essence is to be taken from them all, as the bee takes the essence from many flowers.

इषुकारवन्नैकचित्तस्य समाधिहानिः ॥

One whose mind has become concentrated like the arrowmaker's does not get his meditation disturbed.

कृतनियमलङ्घनादार्थक्यं लोकवत् ॥

Through transgression of the original rules there is non-attainment of the goal, as in other worldly things.

प्रणतिब्रह्मचर्योपसर्पणानि कृत्वा सिद्धिर्बहुकालात्तद्वत् ॥

By continence, reverence, and devotion to Guru, success comes after a long time (as in the case of Indra).

न कालनियमो वामदेववत् ॥

There is no law as to time, as in the case of Vamadeva.

लब्धातिशययोगाद्वा तद्वत् ॥

Or through association with one who has attained perfection.

न भोगात् रागशान्तिर्मुनिवत् ॥

Not by enjoyments is desire appeased even with sages (who have practised yoga for long).

(Book 4)

योगसिद्धयोऽप्यौषधादिसिद्धिवन्नापलपनीयाः ॥

The Siddhis attained by yoga are not to be denied like recovery through medicine etc.

(Book 5)

स्थिरसुखमासनमिति न नियमः॥

Any posture which is easy and steady is an Asana; there is no other rule.

(Book 6)

In Vyasa Sutra

आसीनः सम्भवात् ॥

Worship is possible in a sitting posture.

ध्यानाच्च ॥

Because of meditation.

अचलत्वञ्चापेक्ष्य ॥

Because the meditating (person) is compared to the immovable earth.

स्मरन्ति च ॥

Also because the Smritis say so.

यत्रैकाग्रता तत्राविशेषात् ॥

There is no law of place; wherever the mind is concentrated, there worship should be performed.

(Ch. 4/1)

□□□

LOTUS CHOICES OF INDIA BOOKVARSITY

INDIA BOOKVARSITY is fast growing as the pioneer publishing program of quality works, old and new, on aspects of indian culture, to inform educate and stimulate the new generation and Indiaspora, as also those interested in Indian religions, philosphies, values, etc,. all over the world. **Editor: Mahendra Kulasrestha**

The Golden Books of Indian Religions

Classics Revived for an Ultra-Modern World

In no other country of the world so many religions were born, all peace-loving, with a variety of philosophies, with God and without God, but all believing in Karman and Rebirth. The Buddha's religion was first world movement for peace, kindness and equality, much liked even today. Every educated Indian and others at large should know about them in the present terror-stricken times. The books are specially planned and produced for the general educated reader.

RIGVEDA

The Golden Book of Rigveda: Humanity's Oldest Scripture

—R. T. H. Griffith

The first book of its kind for the general reader.... selected hymns from a very large collection, arranged subjectwise, translated into easy-to-understand English. Griffith's translations of all the Vedas are famous.

ISBN 81-8382-010-7
Rs. 395/

BUDDHISM

The Golden Book of Buddhism: Humanity's Oldest Religion of Peace

— F. Max Muller, T. W. H. Rhys Davids, Samuel Beal

Buddhism is a much-loved and respected religion of modern times which can play a significant role in overcoming terror. Selected suttas, including Ashvaghosa's *Life of Buddha*, translated from its Chinese version, and *Dhammapada*, the *Gita of Buddhism*.

ISBN 81-8382-011-5
Rs. 395/-

JAINISM

The Golden Book of Jainism: Humanity's Oldest Religion of Non-Violence

— Hermann Jacobi

India's unique religion in philosophical analysis and holy practices, more non-violent than any, and much older to Buddhism.

Selections from *Uttaradhyayana Sutra, Acharanga Sutra, Sutrakritanga*, etc., with *Life and Vows of Mahavira*, Simple English.

ISBN 81-8382-014-X

Rs. 395/-

UPNISHAD

The Golden Book of Upanishads: Humanity's Earliest Philosophical Compositions

— F. Max Muller

Proponents of the concepts of Atman, Brahman, Karman, Prana, etc. Much appreciated in the present day world.Eleven major Upanishads as chosen by Shankaracharya, presented in simple English.

ISBN 81-8382-012-3

Rs. 495/

Aspects of Indan Culture

CULTURE INDIA

Culture India: Philosophy, Religion, Arts, Literature, Society

- Ed. Mahendra Kulasrestha

A classic revived. Special contributions by authorities in their respective areas: Dr. Radha -krishnan, Dr. Suniti Kumar Chatterji, Svetoslav Roerich, Ritha Devi, Priya Chatterji Tandura, Dr. A. D. Pusalkar, Prof. K. A.Nilakanta Sastri, etc. etc. etc.

'...encylopaedia of ancient Indian culture.'
- *Journal of American Oriental Society.*

ISBN 81-8382-013-1

Rs. 495/-

RAJAYOGA

Learn RAJAYOGA from VIVEKANANDA

The first easy-to-understand exposition of India's unique philosophy and practice of perfect health and Godhead by the veteran..... which he made for his American disciples. Easily the best and most authentic. With commentary on Patanjali's Yoga Sutra; and Yoga references in *Kurma Purana, Samkhya Karika, Shvetashvatara Upanishad, Shankar Bhashya*, and *Vyasa Sutra*, illustrated.

ISBN 81-8382-009-3

Rs. 395/-

Other Books on

PHILOSOPHY, RELIGION & CULTURE

1. My Experiments With Truth **(New)** 160/-
2. Gandhi Global For The New Gen **(New)** 175/-
3. The Golden Book of World Religions **(New)** 395/-
4. Hindu Social System First Famous Study 295/-
5. The Lotus Sutra Saddharma Pundarika 295/-
6. The Master Swami Vivekananda 250/-
7. Everyman's Book of Hindu Religion & Mythology 295/-
8. The ABC of Hindu Culture 295/-
9. India in China The Gift of Buddha 295/-
10. The Vital Truths of Hinduism 250/-
11. Philosophy India 250/-
12. The Dhammapada 295/-
13. The Last Days of Lord Buddha 295/-
14. Complete Book of Hindu Gods And Goddesses 295/-
15. Vatsyayana's Kamasutra Select and his times 125/-
16. The Kama Sutra of Mallinaga Vatsyayana 125/-
17. Judgment NoAircrashNoDeath 250/-
18. Patriot Netaji Subhas Chandra Bose 250/-
19. The Life of Lord Buddha 295/-
20. The Discourses of Lord Buddha 295/-
21. The Golden Book of Buddhism 295/-
22. The Golden Book of Hinduism 295/-
23. The Golden Book of Islam 295/-
24. The Golden Book of Rigveda 295/-
25. The Golden Book of Jainism 295/-
26. The Golden Book of Upanishads 295/-

27.	Learn Rajayoga from Vivekananda	250/-
28.	Colossus Vivekananda Select	250/-
29.	Intellect India	250/-
30.	Culture India	250/-
31.	Mahatma Gandhi The Bhagavadgita	160/-
32.	Shirdi Sai Baba	80/-
33.	The Ramayana For Every Home **(New)**	125/-
34.	The Mahabharata For Every Home **(New)**	125/
35.	Sai - The Age of Cosmic Family	80/-
36.	Sathya Sai and His Miraculous Powers	95/-
37.	To Bloom Like a Lotus	225/-
38.	The History of Sikh Gurus	225/-
39.	Indian Mythology	195/-

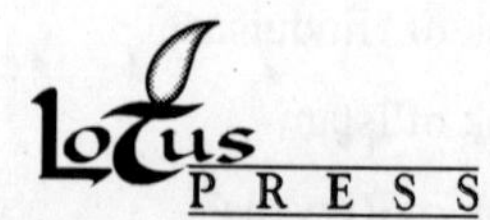

Unit No. 220, 2nd Floor, 4735/22, Prakash Deep Building,
Ansari Road, Darya Ganj, New Delhi- 110002
Ph.: 32903912, 23280047, 9811594448
E-mail : lotuspress1984@gmail.com, www.lotuspress.co.in